The Nurse's Guide to
Writing for Publication

Susan Kooperstein Mirin, R.N., M.S., holds an A.A.S. degree in nursing from the State University of New York Upstate Medical Center in Syracuse, New York, and a B.S. in journalism and M.S. in science communication from Boston University. She practiced nursing for four years, served as editor of *Nurse Educator* for five years and as editor of *The Journal of Nursing Administration* for one year, and has held a variety of other writing and editorial positions. Currently she works as a free lance writer and editor, consults on writing to individuals and groups, and gives writing workshops.

The Nurse's Guide to Writing for Publication

Susan Kooperstein Mirin, R.N., M.S.

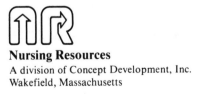

Nursing Resources
A division of Concept Development, Inc.
Wakefield, Massachusetts

This volume was selected for inclusion in the
NURSING DIMENSIONS ADMINISTRATION SERIES
Volume 2, Number 1, 1981
NURSING DIMENSIONS EDUCATION SERIES
Volume 2, Number 1, 1981

Library of Congress Catalog Card Number 80–84085

ISBN 0–913654–71–X   (hardbound)
ISBN 0–913654–73–6   (paperback—subscription edition)

Manufactured in the United States of America

Cartoons on pages 25 and 58 reprinted with permission of
the artist, John Caldwell.

*In Memoriam to my father,
Jacob Kooperstein, who instilled
in me a love of literature and
the desire to write*

Preface

Is writing important to nursing and nurses?

Yes! To keep abreast of change, professionals must share information through writing and publishing. Achieving technical mastery of writing is particularly necessary for health care professionals. As knowledge increases within a specialty, the information to be relayed from one generation to the next grows more complex, demanding growth in the power of individuals to communicate knowledge. In addition, nursing's future position in the health care system depends greatly on how effectively nurses communicate developments within the profession to colleagues, other health care professionals, government and regulatory agencies, and the public. And individual career advancement increasingly depends on writing skills, for professionals who publish receive promotions and other forms of recognition more readily.

Yet even nurses who realize the importance of writing may avoid putting down on paper that article or book prospectus they've been thinking about for months or years. After editing nursing journals for four years, I've drawn two conclusions regarding this reluctance. First, many nurses see themselves as "unable to write" and feel helpless when confronted with the process. Second, they are usually unfamiliar with the mechanics of getting published.

Nurses need access to the special body of knowledge that journalists and other professional communicators draw upon. As these people know, effective writing is a craft to be mastered, not a gift endowed upon a chosen few. This book focuses on writing articles for journal publication, but the emphasis on organization, clarity, and other practical aspects of writing and publishing make it a valuable resource for all writing efforts.

Book authors will find the chapters on outlining, principles of clear writing, illustrations, permissions, and copyright law particularly helpful. Researchers preparing formal research reports can also benefit from the information presented here. However, they may also need to seek out supplemental information regarding the appropriate format for traditional presentation of research data.

Thus, although authors of books and research reports may need additional guidance in specific areas, *all* nurse writers will benefit from *The Nurse's Guide to Writing for Publication*. It tells them how to choose an appropriate topic for a specific journal, write a publishable article, and understand each step of the publishing process.

Acknowledgments

I want to pay special tribute to Steven, Jonathan, and Daniel for their patience and support during those months when I stole many family hours to labor over this book.

In addition, my thanks to my mother, Anna Kooperstein, for her encouragement throughout this endeavor.

Carol Wolfe, nursing editor at Grune and Stratton, Inc., New York City, deserves a particular note of appreciation for her able and thorough assistance with the chapter on copyright law.

I also want to acknowledge the help and support of certain faculty members in the journalism department at Boston University's School of Public Communication: Timothy Cohane, expert writer, gifted teacher, and respected friend, who generously gave me permission to use some of his class materials in this book; Norman Moyes who kept telling me how tough it had been getting *his* book written but somehow he did; Kenneth Tong who helped me get the first chapters off the ground; and Harold Buchbinder whose advice inspired multiple rewrites and a clearer message.

And I want to thank many other friends and colleagues for their encouragement. In particular, I greatly appreciated the patient persistence of my editor, Mark Cowell. And special thanks to Jo-Ann La Spina and Karen Melanson—without their typing skills I doubt that a finished manuscript would have ever emerged.

Contents

Figures

Chapter 1

You *Can* Write a Publishable Article

Don't say you can't write. Anyone who can pass the state board licensing exam in nursing can also learn to communicate effectively via the written word.

Even those of you who hated high school grammar and college composition can, with this book and some effort, produce a clear, well-organized article for publication. If the process is not enjoyable for all, it is not terribly difficult. Don't underestimate yourself! It's simply a matter of learning and applying certain principles. Believe me, it's definitely easier to write a good article than to do your first physical assessment or to apply the nursing process to the care of that eighty-eight- year-old senile patient with multiple fractures and congestive heart failure. And you handle situations like that all the time.

To write that professional article or book, and write it well, you need to know and use principles of clear writing. You'll find them in this book. Applying them may seem difficult at first but will become easier with practice. However, as my progressive nursing fundamentals instructor once said, "You don't have to change fifty dressings to be able to change one right." In other words, your first writing effort can be publishable.

1

As you read this book you will see some examples of excellent writing taken from works of great literature. You may say that a nurse writing for journal publication shouldn't strive for the effect that Hemingway or Tolstoy labored toward. You're right—the purpose of your writing is communication, not art. But the basic principles of good writing apply to *all* writing. Hemingway and Tolstoy merely added another dimension to their ability to communicate effectively. Your article does not have to be imaginative or colorful, although it can certainly benefit from those qualities. But it does have to plainly communicate your message through the mechanisms of logical organization and application of the principles of clear writing.

Don't think that writing for primarily communicative rather than artistic purposes has to be dull. Whether your end product is a novel or a description of a neonatal intensive care unit, the writing process can be creative and interesting. Read this book and apply what you learn. You *can* write that article you've been thinking about—and you can also get it published.

Chapter 2

Choose a Topic and a Journal

What should you write about? Usually you decide to write an article because you have an idea or are involved in a situation that seems important. You think other nurses would be interested in it. However, a topic that is merely interesting is not good enough. Professional journals exist primarily to communicate useful information and to stimulate action. Your topic should have the potential of doing one or both.

It also helps a great deal if you pick a topic that *means* something to you, emotionally as well as intellectually. This isn't always possible—you may be involved in a project your supervisor thinks is important, and even though you find it boring, you're the obvious person to write it up. However, usually *you* choose the topic on which to write, so remember that in writing, as in most things, you're most effective when your heart is in it.

Can you say of your topic, "This is something I think really important?" If not, sit down with a cup of coffee and try to think of a subject with which you would genuinely enjoy tangling. Eventually you will come up with a worthwhile topic or a new angle for the old one that excites your interest[1].

3

It's best to write about subjects you know well. Usually authors of articles for professional journals do write in areas of their expertise. However, it is possible to write certain types of articles, such as a review of the literature, from information gathered from reliable references and experts in the field. If you're passionately interested in a topic, you may research it so thoroughly that your article will be better than that of the expert who fails to consider all points of view.

It always helps if a topic is timely. Editors look for information of high current interest to the profession and for future-oriented content that will help readers cope with forthcoming changes in technology and health care policy. However, most editors also want content that will increase readers' effectiveness in their work. They base editorial decisions on the usefulness of the content to the intended readership.

DETERMINING SCOPE

Consider the scope of your subject. A journal article is not a book. You must limit your topic. For example, if you work with kidney disease patients, you may wish to share your knowledge regarding their care through an article in a nursing practice journal such as *American Journal of Nursing* or *RN*. You have a *lot* to say and decide to call it "Nursing Care of the Patient with Renal Disease." The title has a nice ring to it—but wait—give that topic what I call the "scope test." Ask yourself, "by the time I reach the end of this article, how many major points will I be summarizing?" If your topic receives a score higher than three points you definitely need to limit it. If it scores two or three major points, seriously consider focusing on only one of them. Don't confuse subtopics with major points. Good articles usually make one major point (or have one major theme) that is supported in the article via development of several subtopics. All of the supporting material relates directly to the one major point summarized in the article's conclusion.

The renal disease topic would include many major points or themes. Thorough coverage would probably yield a "scope score" of ten or twenty, for many equally relevant aspects of kidney disease or levels of nursing intervention for kidney patients would need to be dealt with. This topic is appropriate for a book, not an article.

In limiting this topic you might come up with titles such as "Dialysis at Home: The Nurse's Role" or "Watch for the Renal Time Bomb: Urinary Postobstructive Diuresis," the title of a 1978 article published by *RN*[2].

These topics would each score one point on the scope test. In the first, the main point is that the nurse has an important role to play in home dialysis. The different components of that role would be subtopics supporting this theme. In the second article, the one major point is that "careful nursing care is needed to avert a problem that, unwatched and unchecked, could easily prove fatal"[3].

An article can describe several different ways to manage a situation and still get the green light on the scope test. To use another example from *RN,* an article entitled "12 Incredibly Simple Tips on How You Can Control Infection" receives a scope score of one[4]. The twelve tips support the article's one major focus: control of infection.

REVIEW OF THE LITERATURE

At this point you have a relevant and useful topic that is reasonably limited in scope. Next question: Has it been covered recently in the nursing literature?

Check the *International Nursing Index* and the *Cumulative Index to Nursing Literature.* If the topic has not been covered recently and you have established a need for the information, then you're ready to match the topic to a journal, as discussed later in this chapter. If you find that the topic has been dealt with during the past few years, look over the articles and see how similar their content and focus is to what you expect to write. You may find that you intend your article to be quite different, or your survey of the literature may inspire a new focus that will be even more significant than the original one. In approaching an editor regarding such an article, you would point out that several articles on this topic have been published, but that your focus is different and significant and why.

On the other hand, if you find the topic has been thoroughly covered in several journals and from every imaginable perspective, give it up. An article on an important, but as yet relatively untreated topic, will have a better chance for acceptance and will contribute to the literature rather than repeat it.

Once you establish the need for an article, go over all the relevant literature and decide what information should be incorporated into it. Most articles need a literature review to place the subject in perspective and to augment the content. As you review the literature, keep thinking about how *your* article can complement or supplement it or how information already published can help support the content you plan. By the time these review notes are finished you should have a very clear idea of your content and approach.

CHOOSING A JOURNAL

Once your topic is defined and you know what ground the article will cover, you need to determine what readership you will direct it to. Sometimes determining the readership comes before or is part of choosing a topic, for one depends on the other. For example, if the person working with kidney patients knew that the journal *Nurse Educator* was looking for articles for inservice educators, she might consider writing an article entitled "Developing an Inservice Education Program to Improve Nephrology Nursing Care." Awareness of a specific market can certainly determine how a potential author focuses a topic.

Most people, however, choose a topic first, based on their interests and expertise. But before actually writing the article, they should determine which journal(s) they are going to approach for publication. The careful choice of the appropriate journal to which to market a specific article is probably the single most important step in getting your article published.

In "Publishing Opportunities for Nurses: A Comparison of Sixty-Five Journals," Joanne McCloskey discusses the importance of choosing the right journal for your article and presents a table synthesizing useful information on the journals in which nurses might publish[5]. This table includes the following: circulation, organizational association, frequency of publication, article word length, manuscript copies required, author payment, reprint policy, length of time for editorial decision and publication following acceptance, number of solicited and unsolicited manuscripts published each year, and percentages of unsolicited manuscripts that are accepted. With McCloskey's permission, this information was updated in September 1979 for publication in this book. The original information was gathered through a questionnaire survey of appropriate journals. In the update, the questionnaire was expanded to include questions about each journal's referee status and the mailing address for query letters and manuscripts. To determine referee status, journal editors were asked, "Is your journal refereed? (Do experts in a particular field review manuscripts and provide input to editorial decisions?)"

The request for updated information was mailed to the sixty-five journals cited in the 1977 *Nurse Educator* article plus four new journals: the *Journal of Emergency Nursing, Research in Nursing and Health, Nursing Leadership,* and the *Journal of Psychiatric Nursing* and *Mental Health Services.* Forty-two responses were received.

Eight envelopes were returned marked "not deliverable"— readers should investigate the accuracy of the given address and the viability of these journals before mailing manuscripts to them. They are *Hospital Formulary Management, Hospital Forum, Family Health, Inservice Training, Education and Nursing Care, Hong Kong Nursing Journal, Australian Nursing Journal,* and *World Hospitals.*

The most current information on each journal, derived either from the original 1977 survey or the 1979 update is presented in an appendix to this book. An asterisk (*) marks each journal from which updated information was obtained through its editor's response to the 1979 survey update as well as those newer journals first surveyed in 1979. Absence of an asterisk indicates that the information was obtained in the 1977 survey.

In encouraging nurse authors to make use of the information she originally developed, McCloskey wrote, "The process of becoming familiar with the many available journals is time-consuming and many authors simply settle for a choice from the few they know best. Such a practice no doubt leads to the rejection of many good manuscripts: well-known journals are so popular that stiff competition forces a high rejection rate; and specialized journals have such a narrow focus that if your topic is not in their field it will not interest them. Selecting a journal knowledgeably from a wide field reduces such hazards and improves your chances for publication"[6].

Thus, it is vital to your publishing future to choose your topic carefully, focusing it to meet the needs of a specific journal.

NOTES

1. Trimble, J. R., *Writing with Style: Conversations on the Art of Writing* (Englewood Cliffs, N.J.: Prentice-Hall, 1975), p. 6.
2. Tichy, A., and Marchuk, J., Watch for this renal time bomb: urinary post-obstructive diuresis. *RN* 41(11):53, November, 1978.
3. *Ibid.,* p. 56.
4. Fisher, P. C., _____ 12 (at least) incredibly simple tips on how you can control infection. *RN* 41 (November, 1978): 57.
5. McCloskey, J. C., Publishing opportunities for nurses: a comparison of 65 journals. *Nurse Educator* 2(4):4-8, July-August, 1977.
6. *Ibid.,* p. 4.

Chapter 3
Query the Editor

The query letter. What is it? What is it for?

A query asks an editor's interest in reviewing a specific manuscript.

Using query letters is a strictly observed game rule among most experienced nonfiction free-lance writers and commercial magazine editors. This is no accident. Financial survival for many of these writers depends on the volume of articles they sell, and they have found that querying is efficient. As a result every book on writing and selling nonfiction articles has its query letter chapter, and the writing magazines run regular "how-to's" on the topic.

Nurses and others writing for professional journals, as well as their editors, can learn from this tradition. For the well-written query has proved to be a manuscript screening tool that saves time for both writers and editors.

Many nursing journal editors already welcome queries and have immediate respect for the author of a good one. However, this is not a universal phenomenon, and you should review a publication's manuscript guidelines to see if the editor encourages queries. A few years ago at a writing seminar I heard a nursing editor say that she didn't like to have queries, abstracts, or outlines submitted for review. She felt she could only make a decision based on review of the entire manuscript. However, it's possible that she could *reduce* her workload considerably by only screening manuscripts which had potential for her journal, as indicated by an earlier query letter.

Very often, a policy of reviewing only finished manuscripts costs everyone time, to say nothing of mailing fees. Instead of wading through dozens of twenty-to thirty-page manuscripts while authors wait weeks for replies, editors can quickly review a few days accumulation of query letters. With a little experience they are able to immediately screen out those that they have no interest in pursuing and pair them with a firm but friendly form rejection letter. Editors can always scribble a few lines on the form letter should they wish to channel the manuscript to another journal or offer some advice to the author.

Thus, for authors, a major advantage of the query letter system is that they usually learn quickly if an article idea is not feasible for a particular journal and can immediately query elsewhere.

HOW MANY QUERIES AT A TIME?

As an author you are within your rights to simultaneously mail several queries regarding the same article to different journals. You can then pick and choose from those expressing interest. However, it is *not* permissible to send out copies of full manuscripts to several editors. There is an unwritten code between writers and editors that a writer awaits a decision from one editor before sending a manuscript to another. This ethic is based on the time it takes for an editor (and sometimes an editorial advisory board) to review a manuscript and reach a decision. Editors are rightfully angry if, after a time-consuming review process, they accept an article only to have the author write back that it's going to the journal down the street.

Because query letters take far less editorial review time, editors are fairly unperturbed at mass query mailings. However you should realize that if the query is a big hit, you must then write back to three or four editors to tell them the manuscript is going elsewhere. They won't be thrilled. And when your next query arrives these editors may experience an acute drop in desire for *that* article.

Since the response to a query is usually quite prompt, I recommend querying one carefully chosen journal at a time. Always send original letters, not copies, and have one ready to go at all times, should a "does not meet our editorial needs" come in. One query may need to vary somewhat from another anyway, depending on a journal's focus.

QUERIES AND THE EDITORIAL PROCESS

After the initial screening of queries described earlier, editors carefully scrutinize those not immediately eliminated. They look at the proposed content in light of its significance to the readership and the topics required for editorial balance in future issues. Editors also look at the organization and readability of the letter to assess the author's writing ability. This review may result in the rejection of a few more queries.

Since the remaining letters are fairly well-written descriptions of topics of interest, the editor sends each author a note expressing a desire to review the completed article. This letter is only a commitment to *review* the article; it does not indicate acceptance. The note can range from a form letter to a fairly lengthy personal letter with suggestions related to the article's development. Although such input takes some editorial time, many editors find it saves them hours later because the submitted article needs less revision and copy editing. Editors will usually only take the time to make such suggestions if they are very interested in the article.

This is one reason you should send out that query as soon as the idea for an article germinates and the preliminary research is done, rather than wait until the whole manuscript is written. An editor's feedback can be very useful, and it is much easier to integrate developmental suggestions into a gestating manuscript than a finished one.

Another reason for querying is that it's much less painful to have a query rejected than to get a fat manuscript returned in the mail. It may be disappointing to find out that several editors are not interested in your idea, but at least you haven't spent months developing it into an article.

HOW TO WRITE A QUERY

Now you know what a query letter is and why you should write one. What makes a good query? How do you put on one page all the information editors need to figure out that *your* article would make a significant contribution to the nursing literature in general and their journal in particular?

Preplanning

Research both your subject and your publishing market before you write a query. The content must indicate that you know the subject thoroughly. Then, in order to focus the letter correctly, analyze the journal's audience and the usual content. Appendix I overviews most of the journals nurses might publish in. After you choose the journal(s) most appropriate for your topic, you need to review a few recent copies and look over its (their) manuscript guidelines. Your query must show that the article you are planning will suit a journal's editorial style and specific audience.

Organization

I recommend organizing the query according to the "train-of-thought" method described in the August 1969 issue of *Writer's Digest*[1]. This approach has four parts: the snowplow, locomotive, train of cars, and caboose (see figure 1).

The snowplow is a lead paragraph or two that catches the editor's interest and lures him into reading on. (For more information on writing leads see chapter five.) The following paragraphs are two snowplows that hooked me on articles.

Example 1

A cyanotic *black* client looks different from a cyanotic *white* client. We all agree with that statement. We also agree that it is often vital to a client's welfare that the nurse immediately recognize pallor, cyanosis, echymosis and other color changes that indicate changes in physical state. However, many nurses can't

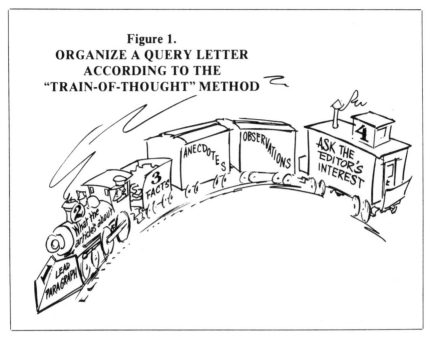

Figure 1.
ORGANIZE A QUERY LETTER
ACCORDING TO THE
"TRAIN-OF-THOUGHT" METHOD

From Henry, O., and Handley, C.A., A four point system for writing a selling query letter. *Writer's Digest,* 49(8):48–51, 1961. Reprinted with permission.

recognize color-related symptoms when they occur in dark-skinned persons [2].

Example 2

CARDIAC ARREST! Just seeing it in print starts the adrenalin flowing. The staff nurse is ready, or is she? Will fear stop her in her tracks? Will she even consider running away instead of rushing to assist? The answer is NO!—if she is properly prepared [3].

After the snowplow you write the locomotive—a paragraph that tells *what* the article will be about. It should point out what direction the article will take and what it will offer the reader. Here's the locomotive that followed the first snowplow cited.

Figure 2.   An Example of a Well-written Query.

November 22, 1978

Susan Mirin
Associate Publisher
NURSE EDUCATOR
607 North Avenue
Wakefield, MA 01880

Dear Ms. Mirin:

A cyanotic black client looks different from a cyanotic white client. We
all agree with that statement. We also agree that it is vital to a
client's welfare that the nurse immediately recognize pallor, cyanosis,
echymosis and other color changes that indicate physical state. However,
many nurses can't recognize color-related changes when they occur in dark-
skinned persons.

It is the responsibility of nursing educators to teach their students physiological assessment of the black person. We are interested in submitting
an article describing how we taught such content to beginning level nursing
students at the University of Michigan. A skin color change assessment
guide is included. The article is written in an informal, narrative style
and several specific clinical examples are included.

This article is important because as nurses take greater responsibility for
client outcomes, it becomes essential that they have the knowledge needed
to provide optimum care to all clients. In addition to providing educators
with necessary information and a framework for teaching it, the article
will help them to facilitate students' sensitivity to the emotional and
cultural needs of the black patient.

In addition, it is hoped that this article will stimulate educators'
interest in developing better understanding of the complete health-related
needs of other racially/culturally different groups.

The rapidly changing health care delivery system demands that nurses become
aware of the characteristics and needs of all races and cultures. This
manuscript can be submitted within one month of receiving your positive
response. We are looking forward to hearing from you.

Sincerely,

Bobbie Bloch, R.N., M.S.

Mary Hunter, R.N., M.S.

Published with permission of the authors.

It is the responsibility of nursing educators to teach their students physiological assessment of the black person. We are interested in submitting an article describing how we taught such content to beginning level nursing students at the University of Michigan. A skin color change assessment guide is included. The article is written in an informative narrative style and several specific clinical examples are presented.

It's not unusual to spend several hours writing and rewriting a snowplow and locomotive. The time invested is worthwhile. Not only does it often result in an editor's positive response to your query, but you can almost always use the snowplow and locomotive as the opening paragraphs of your article. A basic rule for writing snowplows and locomotives is to keep them short; each should be under seventy-five words.

After the snowplow and locomotive you give some facts or observations to back up your premise. These additions are the "cars" in your "train-of-thought." Notice the cars in figure 2, an example of a well-written query[4].

If you have special credentials for writing this article, the last car might state what they are. However, be brief. No editor wants to know that you always liked to write or that you were editor of your high school newspaper. Often merely giving your title after your name and using the stationery of your employing institution will be enough to establish your credibility. Use such stationery whenever possible. If it's not available tell the editor briefly who you are and why you are qualified to write the article.

The last two paragraphs are the caboose. Here you ask the editor's interest in the article and point out when the article could be ready. You also make a strong statement designed to convince the editor that this is an article that should be published.

When your query is written, check it for the elements cited in figure 3.

The importance of displaying good writing skills in the query letter can't be emphasized enough. The letter must be clear, well-organized, and interesting in order to convince the editor that you can write an article with the same characteristics. If possible, limit your query to one single-spaced page.

Figure 3.   Check Your Query.

Increase your query's chances for success by checking it against the six W's.

1. WHAT? Is the article clearly and definitely described? Did you point out how you plan to approach the material?

2. WHERE? Does your query indicate that you know where you're sending it? Does it show that you're aware of the journal's needs, format, readership, editorial policies, and style as reflected in recent issues?

3. WHEN? Is the proposed content *currently* important to nurses—either because it's tied to recent developments or because it's information that doesn't lose its timeliness?

4. WHY? Will editors automatically grasp the importance of your topic? If not be sure to convince them.

5. WHO? Who are you? Indicate any special qualifications you have for writing this article. Are you particularly well qualified because of your personal expertise and access to specific resources? If you don't have great credentials say nothing; let the idea speak for itself.

6. The WAY? *Competently.* Neat typing, correct grammar and sentence structure, accurate information, and perfect spelling.
    Do it: *Concisely.* One page *is* better than two.
    Colorfully. Use intriguing facts or anecdotes to hold editors' attention. Make them want to see more.

GUESS THE EDITOR

The array of editors listed on a professional journal's masthead often leaves an author guessing who might be least surprised at the arrival of a query on his/her desk. Check the journal's manuscript guidelines for the person to whom manuscripts and queries should be sent. In addition to these detailed guidelines, available on request, journals sometimes publish brief instructions to authors somewhere in the publication. You can also call the journal and ask a secretary for the appropriate editor's name. If you can't come up with a name by these methods, send the query to the person listed as editor, associate editor, or editorial director. You don't usually send it to the publisher or managing editor. And contributing editors or editorial advisers are consultants to the journal. Don't send manuscripts or queries to them.

Give the editor fifteen working days to answer your query. If you don't have a response by this time, send a letter asking about the query. State the date of transmission and briefly describe the content.

If an editor expresses interest in reviewing the manuscript for possible publication, immediately acknowledge the letter stating when the manuscript will arrive and responding to any questions.

Overall, editors of nursing journals are becoming increasingly aware of the advantages of the query system and will usually welcome the well-written query.

NOTES

1. Henry, O., and Handley, C. A., A four point system for writing a selling query letter. *Writer's Digest* 49(8):48-51, 1969. Adapted with permission.
2. Bloch, B., and Hunter, M., Query letter submitted to *Nurse Educator,* November 2, 1978. Published with permission of the authors.
3. Prowant, Y., and Stratford, T., Query letter submitted to the *Journal of Nursing Administration,* January 10, 1979. Published with permission of the authors.
4. Bloch and Hunter, 1978.

BIBLIOGRAPHY

Guarine, V. How to learn what editors want and then write the article query. *Writer's Digest,* 48(4):27-40, 1968.
Hallstead, W. F. How to write a query letter. *Writer* 89 (August 1976):23-25.
Jones, I. S. How to effectively query the editor. *Writer's Digest* 55(6):28, 1975.
Moyes, N. D., and White, D. M. *Journalism in the Mass Media.* Lexington, Mass.: Ginn and Co., 1974, pp. 55-56.
Pesta, B. Writing the query letter. *Writer* 88 (July 1975):15-18.

Chapter 4

Develop a Detailed Outline

Outline! Outline! Outline! Outlining is the key to organization. And organization, that most important aspect of clear writing, is often the biggest problem in manuscripts submitted to nursing journals.

The typical poorly organized manuscript jumps from one thought to the next until the reader is dizzy. An editor's usual response is to attach a rejection slip and place it in the "out" box. However, at times a topic is so relevant and the author's expertise so obvious that an editor puts forth a rescue effort. Using the information presented, he/she may spend about fifteen minutes writing a very general outline that organizes the content and send this outline to the author with a request for revision based upon it.

The results are usually amazing. It seems that once authors are aware of the need for organization and the tool for accomplishing it, they can suddenly express their ideas clearly and meaningfully.

Thus the importance of this chapter to your future writing efforts can't be emphasized strongly enough. (For only on rare occasions will editors actually help you reorganize your work.)

WHY OUTLINES WORK

The outline provides an internal order or skeleton for your manuscript that can also serve as a plan for writing it.

Many people abhor outlines; they remember earlier school experiences where outlining was taught and required. Many students regularly completed the assigned writing project and then wrote an outline from it. I know I did. But at this point in your professional career it's time to overcome your past traumatic experiences with outlines. The outline is the sole tool of organization and thus essential to effective writing. Actually, most people find that outlines become objects of dependence and comfort once they start using them. In the midst of a first draft, as note cards, books, and crumpled papers spread across the desk and floor, the outline offers a reassuring sense of order. It's a life raft the writer can cling to in a rising sea of facts, ideas, and statistics.

HOW TO PREPARE AN OUTLINE

With outlines, as with most matters, "if it works, use it!" Hard and fast rules for topic outlines or sentence outlines or combination outlines are unnecessary. As long as an outline helps you structure your content meaningfully, it's OK. As one writing authority said, "An outline is not a strait jacket, it is a tool: its only real requirement is that it be useful[1]."

Start with the Basics

You are ready to write your general outline when you have done enough research to write a good query letter. Your thinking on the subject is clear. You have a definite idea of the major point(s) you wish to make and the content that will support it (them).

When you reach this stage in your preliminary research, write the query letter, a process that will further clarify your thinking. (In order to write an effective query you may have to roughly outline the subject matter first.) Once a positive response to the query is received, I recommend developing your outline in more detail. If that idea frightens you, start out with an outline that one author says is

"as simple to construct as a ham sandwich"[2]. The basic ingredients of a ham sandwich? Two slices of bread and the ham. An outline also has only three basic parts[3]:
  I. Introductory statement
 II. Supporting evidence or details
III. Conclusion

Develop It in Detail

Now you garnish your sandwich. The introductory statement can come plain or with mayo—one paragraph or three or four. The ham is the mainstay: it can come in several layers and with extra ingredients.

Thus, to begin with, get everything you want to include in your sandwich (or article) into the most functional order possible—the way you envision the whole package most effectively presented. At this stage consider the advice from another authority who said that an outline "allows an author to lead a reader by the shortest path to the information he needs"[4].

After you have integrated everything you want to include into the outline, sit back and review it. Outlines always need some revision. Check to see if your basic parts (you'll probably have more than three by now) are at equal levels of importance. Other level entries should also be at the same level of importance (see figure 4). For practical reasons, when writing an article of about twenty pages, I take the most care in developing *in detail* the first few levels of the outline (I, A, I). Subtopics falling lower than the third or fourth level will probably be fine points in the finished article and can be indicated by just a word or two in the outline to remind you to include them.

Revising It

Your outline is a tool, not a strait jacket. It should provide you with a sense of the most effective internal order for expressing the content you need to communicate. But you will almost always revise and adapt it as new ideas and facts crop up.

Double-space the outline and leave four or five spaces between the major headings. Then, as new material appears, you can put appropriate subtopics into place. If major headings need to be changed around, cutting and pasting may be in order. Thus, base your outline on preliminary research and then revise and adapt it to include new material.

Figure 4.   Levels of Importance in an Outline.

I. The first major topic   First level of importance
  A. A subtopic of *I*   Second level of importance
    1. A subtopic of *A*   Third level of importance
    2. A subtopic of *A*
    3. A subtopic of *A*

  B. A subtopic of *I*   Second level of importance
    1. A subtopic of *B*   Third level of importance
    2. A subtopic of *B*
      a. A subtopic of *2*   Fourth level of importance
      b. A subtopic of *2*
        (1) A subtopic of *b*   Fifth level of importance
        (2) A subtopic of *b*
           (a) A subtopic of *(2)*   Sixth level of importance
           (b) A subtopic of *(2)*

II. The second major topic   First level of importance
  A. A subtopic of *II*   Second level of importance
  B. A subtopic of *II*

From C.J. Mullins, *A Guide to Writing and Publishing in the Social and Behavioral Sciences.* New York: John Wiley and Sons, Inc., 1977. Reprinted with permission of John Wiley and Sons, Inc.

Express a Full Idea

Let each topic and subtopic express a full idea. Ideas and relationships among them will be clearer than if one or two word topics are used. For example, in outlining this book, the major heading for this chapter was not "Outlining," but "Develop a Detailed Outline." When it was time to write this section, several weeks after the outline was completed, the phrase provided direction to the work at hand.

Thus, if you outline, organization should not be a problem. Remember that even the most experienced professional writers rely on this tool of organization.

NOTES

1. Ward, R. R., *Practical Technical Writing* (New York: Alfred A. Knopf, 1968), p. 56.
2. McKee, J. D., The writer's all-purpose tool, in F.A. Dickson, (ed.), *Writer's Digest Handbook of Article Writing* (New York: Holt, Rinehart, p.31)
3. Ibid, p. 106.
4. Jordan, J., *Using Rhetoric* (New York: Harper & Row, 1965), p. 106.

BIBLIOGRAPHY

Goeller, C. *Writing to Communicate.* New York: Mentor Executive Library (The New American Library, Inc.), 1974.
Mullins, C.J. *A Guide to Writing and Publishing in the Social and Behavioral Sciences.* New York: John Wiley and Sons, 1977.

Chapter 5

Now Write The Article

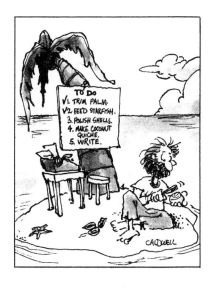

You're ready to write. Your first query letter impressed an editor who gave you a submission deadline three months from today. You spent four evenings and all weekend in the library completing your research and developing a detailed outline. You have a fat file of note cards and copies of papers, a stack of books and magazines with markers sticking out of them, an outline scribbled with "keys" to appropriate research materials, and an intense yearning to do *anything* but write. In fact you're thinking of cleaning your oven or wallpapering the attic. Anything but write that article. Now what?

Getting started *is* hard. That's why it's good to have an outline to push off with. Just get going; don't worry about style. Don't be concerned about which part of the article to work on first. If your introduction drags, turn to another section. The important thing is getting some information down so that you feel you've accomplished something when your writing time is up. It makes getting started tomorrow easier.

Different people have different rituals for beginning a writing chore. One cleans up the work area, rearranges notes, makes a fresh pot of coffee, and polishes an apple or two before touching a pencil. Another sits right down at a typewriter, spreads notes about, and types paragraph after sequential paragraph. Another dives into the job longhand, skipping from one area to the next as thoughts flow. Still another paces the room with a dictaphone, rapidly turning notes and ideas into sentences and paragraphs.

As you do more and more writing you'll settle into a working style comfortable for you, and the process of beginning to write may get easier.

Basically, *don't worry* if you have trouble getting started; it's a universal syndrome. But you do have to start. So exert some self-discipline and grumble your way through the first few hours—tomorrow will be easier.

STUDY THE PUBLICATION AND MANUSCRIPT GUIDELINES

You reviewed the journal and its manuscript guidelines when choosing it and developing your query letter and outline. Study them again as you start writing, concentrating on style. If your article fits the journal, its chance of acceptance will be higher. Look through several back issues and try to get a definite feel for the level of the readership. For a journal that is clinically oriented, ask yourself if most of the content is directed toward new graduate staff nurses or toward inservice educators with master's degrees. Each group requires a different approach. Note whether a certain writing style (such as narrative or question and answer) dominates the articles. See if the journal uses charts, photographs, or other illustrations. Review the manuscript guidelines again to see exactly what the editor expects in terms of illustrations and article length.

location (off-line). You can receive off-line printouts through the mail within a few days.

Charges vary widely by data base, but in general you will pay for the time you are hooked up to the computer by the minute. Additionally, you are charged by the citation for both on- and off-line printouts. It is usually considerably cheaper to choose off-line printouts.

MEDICAL AND HEALTH SCIENCES

1. BIOETHICSLINE—provides bibliographic information on questions of ethics and public policy in health care and biomedical research. Created by the Center for Bioethics, Kennedy Institute, Georgetown University. References date from 1973.
2. CANCERLIT—more then 150,000 references on all aspects of cancer research and therapy, dating from 1963.
3. CANCERPROJ—information on recently completed and ongoing cancer research, from the Smithsonian Science Information Exchange.
4. EXCERPTA MEDICA—comprehensive index to international literature on medicine and related sciences, from 1975.
5. HEALTH PLANNING AND ADMINISTRATION—covers health care planning, organization, financing, management, manpower, and related subjects from 1975.
6. HISTLINE—includes the history of medicine and related sciences, professions, individuals, institutions, drugs, and diseases. Produced by the National Library of Medicine. References from 1970.
7. INTERNATIONAL PHARMACEUTICAL ABSTRACTS—provides information on all aspects of the development and use of drugs and on professional pharmaceutical practice. Created by the American Society of Hospitals, dating from 1970.
8. MEDLINE—files correspond to *Index Medicus*, covering clinical medicine, all areas of medical research, biochemistry, virology, nutrition, and bioengineering. Produced and supported by the National Library of Medicine. References date from 1966.
9. PHARMACEUTICAL NEWS INDEX—covers the four major weekly drug industry newsletters, contains latest information affecting the drug industry, such as major health bills and court actions. References date from 1974.
10. TOXLINE—indexes published human and animal toxicity studies, environmental pollutants effect, adverse drug reactions, and analytical methodology. Assembled by the Toxicology Information Program at the National Library of Medicine. References date from 1965.

SCIENCE AND APPLIED SCIENCES

1. BIOSIS PREVIEWS—covers all aspects of the life sciences from both *Biological Abstracts* and *Bioresearch Index*. References date from 1969.
2. SCISEARCH—covers all fields of physical, biological, and medical literature, corresponds to *Science Citation Index* published by the Institute for Scientific Information. Can also retrieve articles citing an author or paper. References date from 1974.
3. NTIS—the complete *Government Reports Index/Announcements* file from the National Technical Information Service, provides abstracts of technical reports of government-sponsored research and development in virtually all areas of basic and applied science. References date from 1964.
4. SAFETY SCIENCE ABSTRACTS—covers international literature in safety science including industrial and occupational, transportation, aviation and

aerospace, environmental and ecological, and medical safety. References date from June, 1975.

MULTIDISCIPLINARY

1. FEDERAL INDEX—indexes federal government activities, including the *Congressional Record, Federal Register,* the *Washington Post,* and presidential documents. References date from 1977.
2. GPO MONTHLY CATALOG—current bibliography of publications from all branches of the government covering all subjects from Congress, departments and bureaus. Produced by the U.S. Superintendent of Documents. References date from 1976.

EDUCATION

1. ERIC—covers *Research in Education* and *Current Index to Journals in Education,* including all related areas of education. References date from 1966.

SPECIALIZED INDEXES AND ABSTRACTS

1. *The Business Periodicals Index*—lists articles by topic in areas of accounting, advertising and public relations, automation, banking, communications, economics, finance and investments, insurance, labor, management, marketing and taxation.
2. *The Education Index*—covers educational periodicals.
3. *International Nursing Index*—compiled in cooperation with the people who produce *Index Medicus,* this index covers nursing literature published in all languages and includes journals, books, dissertations, association publications. It covers all American Nurses' Association (ANA) and National League for Nursing (NLN) publications. Over 150 nursing periodicals and over 250 nonnursing periodicals are indexed.
4. *Hospital Literature Index*—also associated with the *Index Medicus* group, this American Hospital Association publication is published quarterly and indexes nearly 700 journals by subject and author, including appropriate articles from non-health journals such as *Business Week, Harvard Law Review,* and *Fire Technology.*
5. *Hospital Abstracts*—provides abstracts monthly from 45 international journals, by subject and author. Published by Her Majesty's Stationery Office, London, Ministry of Health.
6. *Cumulative Index to Nursing and Allied Health Literature*—covers over 300 international journals, both popular and biomedical, published every 2 months.
7. *Index Medicus*—comprehensive bibliography of the world's medical reviews, serial journals, and selected monographs, published monthly and cumulatively by year. Includes a short catalog of literature searches recently performed that you can obtain free of charge. Also published in an abridged version, which indexes fewer journals and is somewhat more manageable. Produced by the National Library of Medicine. Also see Computerized Literature Searches for further information regarding *Index Medicus* as a resource.
8. *Excerpta Medica*—a series of 43 monthly publications which abstract medical journals by subject, such as gerontology and geriatrics, public health, social medicine and hygiene. Published in English in Amsterdam. (Also see Com-

4. Newspaper research—*The New York Times Index, The Christian Science Monitor Index, The Wall Street Journal Index,* and the index to *The Times of London* will all direct you through the newspaper literature. When doing newspaper research also check (1) library "clipping" files of local newspaper stories (often available at big libraries) and (2) newspaper libraries or "morgues".
5. *The Readers Guide to Periodical Literature*—best known guide to the general magazine literature.
6. *The Biography Index*—quarterly guide to biographical material in periodicals and books.
7. *Who's Who*—biographical information on persons currently prominent.
8. *Dictionary of American Biography*—looking back at figures in American history.
9. *Who Was When? A Dictionary of Contemporaries*—and *The Dictionary of Contemporaries*—place your subject in historical perspective—for example, find out what famous person lived when Florence Nightingale did.
10. *The Congressional Directory*—biographical information on all members of Congress.
11. *Current Biography Yearbook*—compilation of monthly issues of *Current Biography* which feature biographies of contemporary leaders in the arts and sciences. Published by H.W. Wilson Co., New York.
12. *Facts on File*—weekly news digest covering science, medicine, education, sports, and other broad interest areas, indexed by subject, name of person, organization, or country involved.
13. *What They Said In—The Yearbook of Spoken Opinion*—contains quotations appearing in print in the last year from political and professional leaders on significant topics, including medicine and health.
14. *Editorial Research Reports*—6,000-word studies discussing background and prospects for major issues. Four issues per month.
15. *Congressional Quarterly Service*—weekly reports on congressional action.
16. *The Statistical Abstract of the United States*—the annual Bureau of the Census summary of U.S. social, political, and economic statistics.
17. *Historical Statistics of the United States*—allows a look at earlier statistics.
18. *International Encyclopedia of the Social Sciences*—16 volumes of man's scientific knowledge.
19. *The Vertical File Index*—a guide to available pamphlets.
20. *Encyclopedia of Associations*—lists hundreds of associations in the U.S., from the American Cancer Society to the most obscure stamp collecting group. Provides membership description, address, name of chief officer, and date and place of next association meeting, if known. Check here for specialized or small associations.

COMPUTERIZED LITERATURE SEARCHES

The following data bases list some of the indexes, abstracts, and information banks available either on- or off-line from computerized information vendors. For a complete listing, as well as names and locations of search services, vendors, and data base producers, check the *Encyclopedia of Information Systems and Services,* published by Gale Research and available as a reference work in many libraries.

A computerized literature search is usually done by a long distance telephone connection to the data base. The computer scans titles and abstracts for key words or names that you request. By carefully selecting your key words, you can quickly get specific references on a very narrow topic. The computer will print out the index entries or abstracts on the searcher's terminal (on-line) or at the central computer puterized Literature Searches for more information on this resource.)

9. *Medical Socioeconomic Research Sources*—guide to current publications in sociology and economics of medicine, including journal articles, theses, books, pamphlets, reports, legislation, unpublished speeches, and selected newspapers, indexed by subject and author. Subjects include economics, education, ethics, international relations, and political science. It also includes a list of books indexed during the year. Published by the American Medical Association, Chicago.

10. *Dissertation Abstracts International*—a two-volume set published monthly listing dissertations from over 310 participating U.S. and Canadian institutions. Volume A covers humanities and the social sciences, which includes sociology, law, and education; Volume B covers science and engineering, including biology and health. Both are indexed by keyword, title, and author, and published by Xerox University Microfilms, Ann Arbor, Michigan.

VERY SPECIALIZED INDEXES AND ABSTRACTS—a partial list of the specialized medical resources available at most nursing and medical school libraries.
1. INDEX OF DERMATOLOGY
2. KIDNEY DISEASE AND NEPHROLOGY INDEX
3. CANCER THERAPY ABSTRACTS
4. CURRENT BIBLIOGRAPHY OF EPIDEMIOLOGY
5. ENDOCRINOLOGY INDEX
6. DIABETES LITERATURE INDEX
7. LEUKEMIA ABSTRACTS
8. PSYCHOLOGICAL ABSTRACTS

DIRECTORIES: People, institutions, and organizations with a health care focus.

1. WHO'S WHO IN HEALTH CARE—lists over 8000 biographical sketches containing the professional backgrounds and achievements of leaders in all health care fields. Published by Hanover Publications, New York.
2. NATIONAL HEALTH DIRECTORY—a directory of national, state, city, and county health officials in the U.S., including Congressional committees, key personnel in federal agencies, organizational charts, and maps of HEW buildings. Contains names, addresses, phone numbers and some photographs. Published by Science and Health Publication, Inc.
3. AMERICAN HOSPITAL ASSOCIATION GUIDE TO THE HEALTH CARE FIELD—provides information on health care institutions, the AHA, organizations, agencies, and educational progress in the health field, national hospital statistics data, and sources of products and services used in hospitals. Published yearly by the American Hospital Association, Chicago, since 1945.
4. DIRECTORY OF NATIONAL VOLUNTARY HEALTH ORGANIZATIONS—describes the purpose, organizational pattern, financing and programs of over 50 national medical organizations and agencies of medical interest, divided by subject. Published yearly by the American Medical Association, Chicago.
5. DIRECTORY OF SOCIAL AND HEALTH AGENCIES OF NEW YORK CITY—offers concise and comprehensive information about public and

nonprofit social and health agencies serving NYC, including national agencies with New York offices. Published by Columbia University Press. Check your local department of social welfare to see if such a publication exists for your area.

6. NATIONAL DIRECTORY OF EDUCATIONAL PROGRAMS IN GERONTOLOGY—information on geriatric research and training programs in 121 AGHE institutions. Published by the Association for Gerontology in Higher Education. Check with other associations for similar publications. (See Encyclopedia of Associations.)

STATISTICS (WITH A FOCUS ON HEALTH CARE)

1. FACTS ABOUT NURSING—provides fundamental nursing statistics—demographics, education, economics of nurses and allied health personnel. Published by the American Nurses' Association, Kansas City, Missouri.

2. HEALTH RESOURCES STATISTICS—contains current and comprehensive statistics on a wide range of health areas, including manpower, inpatient, outpatient, and non-patient health facilities, presented in tabular form and organized by state where possible. Published yearly by the U.S. Department of HEW, Office of Health Research, Statistics and Technology since 1965.

3. STANDARD MEDICAL ALMANAC—first published in 1977, provides statistical and narrative data gathered from government and private sources, its five parts cover manpower, income and expenditures, education and licensure, facilities, and disease and disability. Published by Marquis Academic Media.

4. ALLIED MEDICAL EDUCATION DIRECTORY—includes statistics and studies information, problem areas, the accreditation process, and programs by occupation and state. Published by the American Medical Association, Chicago.

5. COMMONWEALTH OF MASSACHUSETTS HEALTH DATA ANNUAL—provides population and vital statistics, health manpower, hospital, home health agencies, preventive medicine, and health financing information for Massachusetts. Published by the Office of State Health Planning. Check your state's Office of Health for similar publications.

GOVERNMENT INFORMATION SERVICES (or, You Might As Well Get Something For Those Tax Dollars)

Every month the Government Printing Office (GPO) publishes the *Monthly Catalog of U.S. Government Publications,* which contains between 1500 and 3000 new entries from federal offices, departments, and agencies. The information and illustrations are not copyrighted. Catalogs are available from the Superintendent of Documents, Washington, D.C. 20402 (202/783-3238) and in most libraries. Some of the publications offered are free, others go for varying, but very reasonable, charges.

In addition, you have free access to federal publications through the Federal Depository Library System, which includes over 1,300 libraries. Many university, state capital, and large city libraries are part of this system. Check with your local librarian for the location of your nearest federal depository library.

The National Library of Medicine is located at 8600 Rockville Pike, Bethesda, MD 20209. There are also eleven Regional Medical Libraries. Check the front of *Index Medicus* for the one in your area.

Compiled by **Ann L. Zevnik,** a science writer and library fixture in Boston, Massachusetts.

WORK FROM YOUR OUTLINE

I'm assuming that you converted to outline use after reading chapter four, and that you developed a detailed outline for your article. This book doesn't provide step-by-step instruction on conducting library research or otherwise obtaining needed facts and opinions. However, to provide some assistance in the information retrieval process, figure 5 lists and describes basic resources for library research with an emphasis on health-related literature.

In addition, here's a basic method for conducting library research and converting the results into a coherent whole.

Develop a general outline leaving wide spaces to accommodate insertions or changes resulting from data collection. As you explore your resources, put source information on 3-x-5 cards coded to correspond to 5-x-8 cards that contain notes with appropriate page numbers. If you make copies instead of taking notes, code the copied pages to the source (3-x-5) cards. As you research, also code the 5-x-8 cards, copied pages, or other materials to your outline so that the accumulated information matches subsections of the outline. When starting to write, organize your notes and then work from the outline. Because all your information is coded to the outline, you can readily find the information you need for each subsection.

Your first draft should be an attempt to "get it all down" as completely and sequentially as possible. In subsequent drafts, concentrate on applying the principles of clear writing discussed later in this

(Text continues on p. 29.)

Figure 5. Writing Resources

Here are some places to look for that information you need. The emphasis is on resources related to health care.

GENERAL INFORMATION

1. *American Library Directory*—a guide to possible sources—it lists libraries with information on their subject areas and special collections.
2. Encyclopedias—Americana, Britannica, Collier, and Grolier cover general information.
3. Almanacs—*Information Please, The World Almanac,* and *Reader's Digest Almanac* contain almost all the facts you would ever want to know.

Fold out

chapter and polishing up details. You usually need to revise the article at least two or three times, and often four or five revisions prove necessary.

If you have access to a typist, you can save time by dictating your marked-up drafts and having them typed double- or triple-spaced. Some people dictate first drafts. Others find working with a pad and pen more effective at that stage.

BEGINNINGS

The writing principles discussed later in this chapter apply to all parts of your article. But certain sections require special attention. The following information will help you write effective titles and lead paragraphs.

The Title

The first words to catch your readers' eyes may represent your final input to the article. Although many writers "name" their creations early in the process, a good title often remains elusive, dancing just out of reach of the writer's consciousness. The right words just don't seem to come together.

In choosing a title remember that it needs to accurately describe what happens in the article in as few words as possible, and at the same time arouse readers' interest. A title's accurate reflection of article content is not only an aid to readers, but also helps future library researchers to find the information they are seeking through indexes and guides to the literature. (If you pick a jazzy title that doesn't indicate what the article is actually about, the article will still be indexed accurately. Writers preparing guides to the literature look beyond the title in determining how to index an article. But persons seeking information through an index may pass your article by if the title isn't keyed to the article's main idea.)

Sometimes you can provoke interest and provide needed information by using the formula, "Catchy Idea of Article: Accurate Reflection of Content," or vice-versa. See how this works in the following examples:

"Comeback from Disaster: Helping the Stroke Patient to Help Himself"[1]

"Faculty Development: Not Just a Bandwagon"[2]

Another mechanism for creating a tantalizing title is the superlative technique. For example, an article about multiple sclerosis might be titled "The World's Most Mysterious Disease." To improve this title for indexing purposes call it, "The World's Most Mysterious Disease: Multiple Sclerosis."

The interrogatory title also catches editors' and readers' attention. An article for nurses on ethical issues in health care might be called, "Should You Ever Refuse a Doctor's Order?" Another article might read, "Is Objective Clinical Evaluation Possible?"

You'll make your article sound exciting and timely if you phrase the title in the active voice. Create a sense of urgency and excitement through titles like, "Reduce Stress on the Job—Now! or "Reach Out to Aging Patients."

Another title trick is the "think negative" heading. See if this formula fits your article. An article about continuing education might be called "You Can Never Afford to Stop Learning." One discussing political issues in health care could be headed "What You Don't Know about Health Care in America". The theory behind this gimmick is that the words *not* and *never* have a certain shock value that jolts the reader and creates interest in the article's content.

You can also scan the Bible, Shakespeare, *Bartlett's Quotations,* everyday expressions, and even nursery rhymes to find ideas and directions for titles. For example, I once noticed an article on child abuse called "Wednesday's Child." Or an article on the dynamics operating with clients who consistently overeat might be called "Licking the Platter Clean: The Obsessive Eater." Borrowing from Shakespeare, you might call an article on using consultants "Lend Me Your Expertise."

Use these ideas or combinations of them to create titles that will make editors and readers sit up and take notice.

The Lead Paragraph

In your introductory, or lead, paragraph, you need to catch readers' attention and focus it on your central idea. At the end of the lead or in the second paragraph, tell readers exactly what to expect from the article and "lead" them into it.

Writing a good lead requires effort. You may revise your manuscript three or four times, but you'll often write two dozen opening paragraphs before you're satisfied. However, if you used the query system, you probably wrote your lead already; the first paragraph of a good snowplow (see chapter three) is usually the perfect lead.

All writers, fiction and nonfiction agonize over their leads. Eva Ibbotson, writing about leads in *The Writer's Handbook,* describes the opening sentence as a "seed; ... a promise, something which encapsulates what follows." She tells how Plato wrote the opening sentence of *The Republic* fifty times: "I went down to Piraeus yesterday with Glaucon, the son of Ariston. As this was the first celebration of the festival I wanted to make my prayer to the goddess and see the ceremony"[3].

Plato's opening may not *seem* too striking, but this fiftieth try has a quality which carries readers forward into one of the most influential works ever written.

If you look at the opening paragraph of any great author's work you will see that it resulted from painstaking craftsmanship. Look at Raphael Sabatini's opening to *Scaramouche:* "He was born with the gift of laughter and a sense that the world was mad"[4]. Or the first paragraph of *A Tale of Two Cities* where Dickens declares, "It was the best of times, it was the worst of times, it was the age of wisdom, it was the age of foolishness"[5].

Whether it opens a work of fiction, a news feature story, or an article for professionals, the ideal lead provokes interest, is direct and concise, and makes promises which are later fulfilled.

Nine techniques for developing leads follow. They were among the writing strategies taught in newswriting classes at Boston University's School of Public Communication. Remember, the initial sentences in your lead paragraph need to be "provocative" statements that catch readers' attention and focus it on the article's central idea. Always follow such statements with one or two sentences that tell readers just what the article is about and what they can expect to gain from it.

Techniques for Writing Leads

Type 1: This is important. (The tone of this opening is grave and thoughtful.)

Example

> You may have to care for a patient with a pneumothorax when you least expect it. That's because either spontaneous or tension pneumothorax can frequently occur without warning in patients who have a chronic pulmonary strider. Rarely do they occur conveniently, when the doctor is at the bedside[6].

Type 2: A quote that reflects the article's essence. (One from a famous person or leading authority works well.)

Example

> "The desire to become more and more what one is, to become all one is capable of becoming."
> Thus Maslow described the need for self-actualization. His theory served as the basis for the development of an effective faculty evaluation tool in our baccalaureate nursing program[7].

Type 3: Here is something of unexpected interest. (Notice the tension and eagerness.)

Example

> Obesity—a problem for many people—and a hazard for anyone with cardiac or respiratory disease. But new research offers hope. A nurse researcher believes that the answer to treatment of obesity problems lies in understanding more about mechanisms which underlie feeding behavior and control appetite.

Type 4: There is something mighty wrong here. (This opening indicates that a problem will be explored.)

Example

> The first day after her gall bladder operation, Mrs. Mundy had been alert and cooperative. She was voiding in small amounts and didn't seem to be in too much pain. Still, the fluid from her penrose drain was bloody. Later that day her pulse rate climbed to 136. And still, her urinary output hadn't increased—despite continuous intravenous[8].

Type 5: There's more to it than appears on the surface. (This prose is lightened by its rhythm and words such as streamed, brightened and sun. The idea is to provide a dramatic contrast with the serious content that will follow.)

> Sun streamed through the windows on 3-North and a bowl of yellow daffodils brightened the nurses station as Jane Keen, head nurse, began patient rounds.

Type 6: Relax. You don't have to be serious all the time. (The wording and sentence structure have a suggestion of flippancy.)

Example

Spring. Exams over. Graduation around the corner . . .

Type 7: Now here's the situation I'm in. (The reader is taken into the writer's personal confidence.)

Example

> A month ago I graduated from a top university based nursing program. Now I'm sitting here in my efficiency apartment—just three blocks from the large medical center where I work. It's Friday—the end of my first week in the real world of nursing practice . . . and I'm full of mixed feelings.

Type 8: Here's the way it was. (The reader is placed directly in the situation.)

Example

It was 10 A.M. on Saturday morning and snowing hard. Because of the weather several nurses were unable to get in and our unit, like most of the hospital, was understaffed. The recovery room nurse called to give report on two patients she was transferring to us—both had required emergency surgery during the night, following injury in an auto crash on the snow-slick expressway.

Type 9: What about this? (The reader is asked a question that arouses his curiosity.)

Example

Do your patients want antibiotics for everything, even a cold?

Remember, in your lead paragraph and the one or two that follow you must:

1. Attract and arouse readers' interest in the article.
2. Focus on the central idea of the article.
3. Tell readers exactly what to expect from the article and lead them into it.

In writing the lead you are synthesizing—putting the whole meaning of your article into a few sentences. You are reducing your subject matter to a picture that can be grasped.

HOW TO WRITE CLEARLY

Are you afraid that this chapter and other "how-to-write" books and courses will have you diagramming sentences and shuddering over possessive singulars? Frightening thought. Don't worry; lots of professional writers can't diagram sentences. You won't hear about diagramming or dangling participles or split infinitives in this book. But you will hear some dogmatic advice regarding CLEAR WRITING. The formula for clear writing consists of applying the following ten pieces of advice to writing that is already solidly organized through use of a detailed outline. The interesting thing about this formula is that it works.

1. *Remove all unnecessary words.* This rule may be the most important and the most painful for professionals and academicians to integrate. They often subscribe to the idea that to be judged as worthy they must sound profound as evidenced by the use of a great number of long, complicated words delivered via the most complicated sentence structure ever dreamed possible.

Such writing only confuses readers, but usually no one tells the authors, particularly if they are well known, and known to be intelligent. (Very intelligent people can be *terrible* writers.)

Write to communicate, not to impress. Forceful writing is succinct. For the most part, keep your sentences short. Sentences pruned of distractions communicate best. This doesn't mean that you can't provide detail about a subject, for pertinent detail adds life, completeness, and accuracy to written material. But take out the noncontributors—the words, sentences, and paragraphs that are redundant or add little to the readers understanding of the topic.

2. *Be direct: use familiar, simple words and phrases.* See figure 6 for some instances where a simpler word can often (not always) substitute for a more complicated one[9]. Simpler words usually communicate more clearly than complex ones.

3. *Use the active verb and the active infinitive whenever possible.* Don't say, "A great number of instruments were laid out in rows on the operating room table." Say, "Rows of instruments covered the operating room table."

In a few instances, you are better off using passive voice or the verb *to be,* but most sentences benefit from phrasing that puts the action in the verb.

Maurie Maverick, the late congressman from Texas, called writing with too much passive voice and too many needless words "gobbledygook." He said that government bureaucrats wrote that way to put themselves on record, but their foggy message ensured that no action would result.

The following example of the befuddling effect of both overuse of the passive voice and failure to omit unnecessary words appeared in *Editor and Publisher* and is reprinted here with permission[10]. It originated during a wartime press conference at which President

---

Figure 6.   Substitute a Simple Word for a Complex One.

INSTEAD OF	TRY	INSTEAD OF	TRY
accomplish	do	divulge	say, tell
achieve	do	donate	give
acquire	get	during the course of	during
add an additional	add		
additionally	also		
anticipate	expect	each and every one	each
any and all	any, all	employ	use
appear	seem	endeavor	try
appreciate	be grateful for	equally as	equally
arise	get up	evidence	show
ascertain	find out	experience	feel
assist	help		
as though	if	facilitate	make easy
as to	about, on	for the purpose of	for, to
as to why	why	for the reason that	because
at all times	always		
at the present time	now	forward	send
at the time of	during		
at the time that	while		
at this time	now	general consensus	consensus
be acquainted with	know	had reference to	meant
be associated with	work for (or with)		
be aware of	know		
by means of	with, in, by	if and when	if, when
		in a manner similar to	to, like
calculated to	likely to	in a position to	can
commence	begin, start	in all probability	probably
consensus of opinion	consensus	inasmuch as	because, since
consider	think of	in connection with	in
consult	ask	indicate	show
contemplate	think of	individual	person
continue on	continue	in excess of	more than
contribute	give	inform	tell
		initiate	begin, start
deem	think	in order to	to
desire	want to, wish	inquire	ask
despite the fact that	although	in regard to	about, on
		in relation to	for
determine	find out	in respect of	of

INSTEAD OF	TRY	INSTEAD OF	TRY
in the event that	if	realize	know
in the immediate vicinity of	near	recall	remember
		receive	get
in the majority of	most	refer back	refer
in the near future	soon	regret	be sorry
in the neighbor-hood of	about	relative to	of
		remark	say
in view of the fact that	because, since	render	make
		reply	answer
		require	call for, need
		reside	live
locality	place	response	answer
locate	find	retain	keep
		reveal	show
		rise	get up
make the acquain-tance of	meet		
materially	much	seek	look for
		so as to	so
necessitate	call for	state	say
new innovation	innovation	subsequent to	after
		subsequently	later
		substantially	much
obtain	get	sufficient	enough
on account of the fact that	because		
on behalf of	for	take place	happen
on the order of	about	terminate	end, stop
optimistic	hopeful	thus	so
		to all intents and purposes	so
peruse	read		
place	put	transmit	send
position	job	transpire	happen
possibly may	may		
presently	now	until such time as	until
presume	suppose	utilize	use
previous to	before		
primary	first		
prior to	before	with respect to	about, in to
purchase	buy	with the exception of	except (for)
		would seem	seem
qualified expert	expert		

Franklin D. Roosevelt read the following order concerning black-outs that had been prepared by the director of civilian defense:

Such preparations shall be made as will completely obscure all federal buildings and nonfederal buildings occupied by the federal government during an air raid for any period of time from visibility by reason of internal or external illumination. Such obscuration may be obtained either by blackout construction or by terminating the illumination. This will of course require that in building areas in which production must continue during a blackout, construction must be provided that internal illumination may continue. Other areas, whether or not occupied by personnel, may be obscured by terminating the illumination.

After the press had interrupted the reading of this order with laughter several times, Roosevelt directed that it be reworded:

Tell them that in buildings that will have to keep their work going, put something across the windows. In buildings that can afford it, so the work can be stopped for awhile, turn out the lights.

4. *Use explicit, clear-cut words* that summon up pictures in readers' minds. Using abstract terms makes writing foggy and unmemorable. Which of the following two statements would you remember?

The number of new nurses in the hospital seems to be increasing.
Four new nurses joined the staff yesterday.

The second sentence creates a picture in your mind. You *see* the new nurses. If you have doubt that such writing works, look at the writings of the masters of literature—Shakespeare, Dickens, Dante—their words come together like a camera being focused, leaving the reader with a clear image of the content.

Even when dealing with content that is inherently abstract, such as theoretical concepts or principles, authors must provide specific, picturable examples to illustrate the concepts. "Don't *tell* your readers what you want them to know; *show* them. Make them feel, hear, taste or smell it . . . The more abstract the idea you are explaining, the more concrete your supporting material should be"[11].

5. *Be assertive.* (Yes, you have to be assertive in your writing too!) Hesitant language adds another barrier to readers' understanding.

Which sentence says it best (most clearly)?

I don't remember her ever starting clinical conferences scheduled for 11:30 before or after that time.

She starts clinical conferences at 11:30 sharp.

The second sentence is assertive – and clear.

6. *Use words that accurately reflect your meaning.* The right nouns and verbs are particularly essential to clarity. If you can't arrive at a word that exactly fits your meaning, use a thesaurus to find one that does. (Incidentally, a good thesaurus is probably a writer's chief weapon against weak or inaccurate word usage. It's a good guess that as an author's writing improves, his/her thesaurus becomes increasingly dog-eared.)

Don't think that adjectives and adverbs aren't important. Some powerful pieces of writing have resulted from excellence in their use. But, in general, they don't drive meaning home with the force of the right nouns and verbs.

7. *Use variety freely.* Encouraging you to lean toward short sentences doesn't mean they should *all* be short. They *do* all have to be clear though. Varying the arrangement of words and sentences will help keep your reader interested.

For example, if you have written several sentences that begin with "the" and are straightforward "simple" sentences, you need to introduce some change. Otherwise your paragraph will develop a dull, thumping quality that will inevitably make readers yawn and very likely cause them to put it aside.

Imagine you are writing the following paragraph about the distractions to cope with in running a hospital floor.

The medication for Mr. Jones was due at 7:30 P.M. The patient was in X ray at that time. The nurse called that department. She asked what time he would be sent back to the floor.

A little too "thumping," right?

You might rewrite it, varying the sentence structure, using more active voice, and eliminating unnecessary words.

Mr. Jones needed his medication at 7:30. Since he was in X ray then, the nurse called to see when he would return.

8. *Tie your content to your readers' experience.* To communicate effectively, you need to provide that vital link in the chain between readers' previous experiences and the new information you're providing. Otherwise either they won't understand the content you offer, or, not being aware of its relevance for them, they won't remember it.

For example, if you're writing a piece advocating operating room experience for all nursing students, briefly recount past developments regarding such experience and also relate the topic to your readers' probable experience. You might ask them: "Did you spend time in the O.R. as a student?" And then say,

> Statistics point out that up until 1960 most students did have an O.R. experience. Do you remember yours? Maybe you just remember the anxiety: Would you contaminate something? Would four fingers get stuck in the thumb of the sterile glove? Would an obsessive surgeon yell at you?
>
> But you also saw, and perhaps were part of, a sophisticated interdisciplinary team cooperating intensely for the welfare of a patient. You also saw that proper aseptic technique was a very serious matter, that it could mean the difference between a patient's speedy recovery and a debilitating or fatal secondary infection. You . . .

Successfully relating your content to your readers' past experiences and current knowledge gets them hooked on your article and makes them eager for and receptive to the information.

9. *Use a topic sentence in each paragraph.* The topic sentence expresses the central idea of a paragraph. Experienced writers *can* turn out clear, effective paragraphs without putting down an actual topic sentence for each one, but less skilled writers should plan to build the use of topic sentences into their writing. Doing so helps you to focus your thoughts and also combats the "spineless paragraph" syndrome. If a paragraph doesn't have a topic sentence, be sure that its main idea is obvious to the reader.

Usually the topic sentence comes first in a paragraph. Often it starts out with a transitional phrase, tying it to the thoughts in the previous paragraph. Now and then it comes last or is integrated into the body of the paragraph.

10. *Provide transition: the bridge over all gaps.* Offer transition from thought to thought, sentence to sentence, and paragraph to paragraph thus guaranteeing your reader a smooth passage through your work.

Transitions are the mortar that hold the building blocks of thoughts together in a paragraph or between paragraphs. These thoughts should already "hang together" clearly if they are properly arranged through careful, logical organization. But correct use of transitions will tie them even closer and further enhance the clarity of your message.

How do you provide transition? You usually use one of the following transition words to help create the link you need: *and, but, yet, however, therefore, consequently, moreover, accordingly, and then, again, at the same time, as a result, in the meantime, for example, for instance, on the other hand, first, second, finally, in conclusion, similarly, conversely, in other words.* Pronouns such as *this, that, these, those, his, hers, its,* also provide transition when used so that they carry the reader's thoughts back to previous material.

The appropriate repetition of certain key words—words fundamental to your article—will also help achieve a smooth flow of thought.

Transitions between paragraphs can consist of either connecting words or phrases and often constitute the opening part of a paragraph's topic sentence. Less frequently authors use a full sentence of transition. And once in a while a transition takes an entire paragraph. In addition to following these ten pieces of advice, I highly encourage authors to absorb, inhale, ingest, or otherwise integrate into their consciousness the content of *The Elements of Style* by William Strunk, Jr., and E. B. White[12]. This seventy-eight-page book manages to include all the writing specifics you need to know, complete with vivid examples.

BLOOD, SWEAT AND REWRITE

In the *Ars Poetica* Horace said that if you ever like anything you write, all you have to do is put it in a chest for seven years and when you take it out you will surely burn it[13]. Horace wasn't joking. Rereading your work always reveals a need for improvement. Of course you can't afford seven years. But neither can you afford under three rewrites.

Timothy Cohane, professor emeritus at the Boston University School of Public Communication, turns out students who can write and write clearly. They start out by memorizing *The Elements of Style*. Then they write, and rewrite, and rewrite, and rewrite and . . . It's no wonder he calls his formula for clear writing "Blood, sweat, and rewrite"[14]. Some of Professor Cohane's guidelines for his writing classes are recreated here with his permission. As you read them remember that the specific process he advocates for producing an article (that of writing the first draft longhand while sitting in an easy chair and so forth), does not have to be followed exactly for you to write successfully. It seems to work well for many persons, but you might prefer to dictate your first draft or write it standing up at the kitchen counter. What is important about the process described here is the revision and rewriting that takes place.

On the first day of class Professor Cohane makes his expectations clear as follows:

"Unless you accept my writing philosophy—that of blood, sweat, and rewrite—you're wasting your time here. And remember, the following guidelines are *minimal*.

"When you are ready to write, seek out a comfortable chair—an insularized haven, with your only company your research, references, lined pads and pencils. This is the best way to think and to write, to rethink and to rewrite, to rethink and to rewrite . . .

"You should order your material into a functional outline. Regard that outline as a kind of first draft—in many ways the most important draft. A carefully wrought outline will not guarantee against road blocks or traps in the drafts that lie ahead. But it will reduce them. After you have finished the outline, write the first draft in pencil on lined paper on a pad and put it aside for twenty-four hours. Then go back to the easy chair, edit that first longhand draft carefully and rewrite it in longhand.

"Now—and not until now—go to the typewriter and copy the latest longhand draft. In this first typing you will find yourself editing a bit. But it will be mainly a copying job. It will be, by formal count, the second draft. Put this draft aside for twenty-four, forty-eight, or if you can find the time, even seventy-two hours. Then take it back to the easy chair.

"And now, with a sharp pencil, edit yourself severely. Toughen your ego by giving it a real lashing. Go back to the typewriter for the second time. Again you will find yourself editing a bit, but again it will be essentially a copying job. It will be, by formal count, the third draft and the last for the time being.

"Edit this manuscript carefully for mistakes.

"Throughout this process of thinking and writing, rethinking and rewriting, rethinking and rewriting, remember these guidelines:

1. Eliminate every word not necessary to clarity and grace. This in itself is quite a task. The best pro who ever lived couldn't escape it.

2. Check all verb forms to make certain you've used the active voice and the active infinitive as often as possible.

3. If the situation calls for the passive, the verb to be, or the participle, OK. Then use it. But examine it as you would a stranger at the door; certify its credentials.

4. Be especially wary of the participle, especially the present participle. Next to verbosity, it seems to be the student writer's most recurrent malady.

5. Check your paragraphs carefully to make sure they are in the right order. Does paragraph six belong up between two and three? Perhaps paragraph eight will make a stronger lead than the one you have. If so, don't hesitate to make the change.

6. Whenever the sequence of paragraphs poses a problem, scissor the pages into paragraphs, rearrange them on the table and number them. This process has been found useful by many successful professionals.

7. Check the sentences within each paragraph to make sure the thoughts are in order. Numbering the sentences is helpful.

8. Check every sentence closely to see if it can be strengthened by placing a name, thought, or word at the end. The story teller doesn't reveal his punch line prematurely nor does the dramatist his denouement. Strength at the end makes the sentence crack like a whip.

9. Strive to make your transitions as smooth and immediate as you can. Just as there is nothing like the active verb to make a story march, race, and explode, there is nothing like the transition to keep it from stumbling. Check transitions not only from para-

graph to paragraph but from sentence to sentence within the paragraph.
10. Use the concrete word instead of the abstract, the familiar instead of the unfamiliar, the picturable instead of the wooden.
11. Be conscious of the value of parallel form. Understand the use of antithesis. But don't overuse them.
12. Don't overuse anything. Without variety, the sound of writing becomes a dull monotonous thumping.

"Above all, in your writing, you must be clear. Clarity doesn't make style but there can be no style without it, and clarity means order. *Without order you cannot communicate. You might just as well sit in the dark and make faces. Or play a coronet in a cave.*"

ENDINGS

The Concluding Paragraph

A strong closing paragraph helps you *twice*. It provides the reader with a final summary of the point(s) made in the article, and it helps to hold the reader, since many people read the opening paragraph, scan the high points and jump to the conclusion. A strong closing encourages them to read the whole piece.

How do you close an article? Several methods work well. You can answer the original question posed. For example, if you start out your lead with a question, you might close by recalling the question and summing up the answer that was provided through the content of the article[15].

Just as you can open an article with a quote, you can summarize a message and leave the reader with a parting thought through the use of quotes. For example, an article on the need for nurses to make changes in education and practice that will enable the profession to better meet current health care needs, even when such changes mean giving up traditional and comfortable ways, might end with the following well-known passage by Frost.

"Two roads diverged in a wood, and I—
I took the one less traveled by,
And that has made all the difference[16]."

Such a closing adds a universal perspective to nurses' efforts to move the profession forward through innovative and often bold moves into previously uncharted territory.

Overall, an article's conclusion should tie up the important points covered and leave the readers satisfied that the goals established in the early paragraphs have been met.

NOTES

1. Kauchak, M.A., Comeback from disaster: helping the stroke victim to help himself. *Nursing* 79 9(8):32, November, 1979.
2. Hipps, O., Faculty development: not just a bandwagon. *Nursing Outlook* 26(11):692-696, November, 1978.
3. Ibbotson, E., In the Beginning, In Burack, A.S., *The Writer's Handbook* (Boston: The Writer, 1974), p. 87.
4. Sabatini, R., *Scaramouche: A Romance of the French Revolution* (Boston and New York: Houghton Mifflin, 1921).
5. Dickens, C., *A Tale of Two Cities* (New York: Random House, Inc., 1950)
6. Meador, B., Pneumothorax: providing emergency and long-term care. *Nursing 78* 8(11):43, November, 1978.
7. Nash, G., Faculty evaluation. *Nurse Educator* 2(6):9, November, 1977.
8. Kurtz, K., Kempema, J., and Birnbaum, M.L. Caring for the patient with acute abdominal crisis and more: multisystem failure. *Nursing 78* 8(11):24, November, 1978.
9. Ward, R.R., Fog and How to Fight It, In Ward, R.R., (ed.), *Practical Technical Writing* (New York: Alfred A. Knopf, 1968), p. 70.
10. Copperud, R.N., Gobbledygook, *Editor and Publisher* November 28, 1959, p. 4.
11. McKee, J.D., The Writer's All-purpose Tool, In F.A. Dickson, (ed.), *Writer's Digest Handbook of Article Writing* (New York: Holt, Rinehart and Winston, 1968), p. 107.
12. Strunk, W. Jr., and White, E.B., *The Elements of Style,* 2nd ed. (New York: Macmillan Co., 1972).
13. Horace, *Ars Poetica*
14. Cohane, T., Blood, Sweat, and Rewrite. Unpublished handout to students at Boston University School of Public Communication. Published with permission of author.
15. Goeller, C., *Writing to Communicate* (New York: The New American Library, 1974), p. 105.
16. Frost, R., Stopping by Woods on a Snowy Evening, In Oscar Williams, ed., *The Pocket Book of Modern Verse* (New York: Pocket Books, Inc., 1958), p. 240.

BIBLIOGRAPHY

Bernstein, T. M. *The Careful Writer.* New York: Athenum, 1965.

Burak, A. S., ed. *The Writer's Handbook.* Boston: The Writer, Inc., 1979.

Day, R. A. *How to Write and Publish a Scientific Paper.* Philadelphia: ISI Press, 1979.

Ewing, D. W. *Writing for Results in Business, Government, the Sciences and the Professions,* 2nd. ed. New York: John Wiley and Sons, Inc., 1979.

Kierzek, J. M., and Gibson, W. *The Macmillan Handbook of English.* New York: Macmillan Co., 1963.

King, L. *Why Not Say It Clearly: A Guide to Scientific Writing.* Boston: Little, Brown and Company, 1978.

Kolin, P. and Kolin J. L. *Professional Writing For Nurses.* St. Louis: The C. V. Mosby Co., 1980.

Chapter 6
Illustrations and Tables

Articles always benefit from appropriately used illustrations and tables. Including such items provides a break in the text and can help clarify information for the reader.

ILLUSTRATIONS

Use illustrations to state points more clearly and efficiently than you can in words[1]. The term illustration usually refers to a variety of items including line drawings, paintings, photographs, charts, graphs, and maps. They are generally called "figures" in the text, that is, figure 1, figure 2. Tables are not considered illustrations because they are set in type rather than reproduced from art work[2].

All illustrations should be numbered with sequential arabic numerals, beginning with 1, and they should be referred to in the text by number. Each illustration should be presented on a separate page of the manuscript, and the drawings, graphs, and figures should be clearly made up in black ink. Before spending a great deal of time preparing illustrations, check with the editor to see if the journal's production department normally assists in final preparation. You may be able to submit clear but unfinished sketches that the art department will reconstruct in a professional manner.

At the top of each illustration type its number and title. This is referred to as the illustration's *caption*. Also, at the top of each illustration, write "top" lightly in pencil.

On the reverse side of the illustration write lightly your name, the illustration's number, and a word or two from the manuscript title to identify it.

Refer to each illustration in the text and provide a circled location note indicating where it should appear. For example, "figure 3 about here" would appear at the beginning of the paragraph where you would like the illustration to be inserted.

Usually, *legends* (footnotes or explanations regarding the illustration) appear at the bottom of the figure. The legend should be typed on a separate page, clearly indicating which illustration it refers to. If it is short it can be written or typed on the page with the illustration, but it should also be typed separately to facilitate typesetting.

PHOTOGRAPHS

Photographs are special types of illustrations because they require special handling. Photographs intended for publication should have excellent tone and contrast and be sharply focused. Acceptable sizes range from 5 x 7 to 11 x 14 inches, although no strict rule exists. Snapshot size is usually too small, but check with your editor, because sometimes a snapshot can be used. Most nursing journals use black and white photographs, but if you are interested in submitting color photos, check the manuscript guidelines or ask the editor if the journal can use them. When a journal can accommodate color photographs, editors usually prefer color transparencies ($2^{1}/_{4}$ x $2^{1}/_{4}$ inch slides) rather than prints.

When working with black and white photographs, editors usually like to have 8 x 10s that are printed on glossy paper. All photographs must be captioned and the captions attached to the picture. Do not write on the back of the photos since pressure will mar the picture surface. Instead type your caption, on the bottom third of an $8^{1}/_{2}$ x 11 inch sheet of paper and attach the photograph to the top of the piece of the paper with a small spot of rubber cement on the back of the photograph. Then fold the bottom part of the paper over the front of the photograph. It is also a good idea to label the back of the photograph with a small gummed label with your name and a few words from the title of the manuscript[3].

TABLES

Tables are a useful means of presenting large amounts of detailed information in a small space. A simple table can often give information that would require several paragraphs to present in the text, and it can make the information far clearer. Whenever the large amount of information that needs to be conveyed threatens to bog down the flow of an article, especially when large numbers of individual but similar facts are involved, an author should seriously consider using a table[4].

Some further guidelines for using tables are: (1) if you have more than eight entries and the data would be clearer in a table than in the text; (2) if use of a table will show relationships more clearly than text would; (3) if the use of the table will reduce the amount of discussion needed[5].

In planning a table an author needs to think about whether its physical dimensions will fit within a journal page. A useful rule of thumb is that a table typed in elite type, single-spaced, on 8½ x 11-inch paper with normal margins will just about fill the type area of a 6 x 9 inch printed page when set in eight-point type. In other words, a full-page table typed single-spaced is roughly equivalent to a full-page table set in the usual size type of an average size book. Journal pages are usually a little larger than book pages.

Every table should be given a number and should be cited in the text in the order it appears in the article. A table always has two columns and usually more. Column headings appear at the top, briefly identifying the nature of the material in the columns. These titles are often called "box heads." The left-hand column of the table is called the "stub" (like the stub in some checkbooks). It is a vertical list of items about which information is given in the columns of the table's body.

Tables are sometimes constructed in very complicated ways. Detailed instructions regarding them can be found in *A Guide to Writing* and *Publishing in the Social and Behavioral Sciences* by Carolyn

J. Mullins and *A Manual of Style* published by the University of Chicago Press. See the reference section of this chapter for detailed bibliographic information regarding these and other resources.

Remember that permission must be acquired for the reprinting of any table or illustration published elsewhere. In fact, most illustrations are copyrighted by the creator even if they have not yet been published. A few exceptions exist, so it is useful to check with your editor regarding the need for obtaining permission to use an existing table or illustration in your article.

NOTES

1. Mullins, C., *Writing and Publishing in the Behavioral Sciences* (New York: John Wiley and Sons, 1977), p. 40.
2. *A Manual of Style,* 12th ed. (Chicago: University of Chicago Press, 1969), p. 225.
3. Ellinwood, L., and Moser, J., *Writer's Market '72* (Cincinnati: Writer's Digest, 1971), pp. 13-14.
4. *A Manual of Style,* p. 273.
5. Mullins, *Writing and Publishing,* p. 34.

Chapter 7
References and Permissions

By the time you receive your R.N., you've written enough papers to know how to reference material from other sources. If you do need a quick review, several excellent sources of information on referencing exist; a few are listed at the end of this chapter. In addition, always follow a specific journal's manuscript guidelines regarding appropriate reference format.

However, when writing for publication, in addition to knowing *how* to reference you need to know *when* quoting from another work requires permission of the copyright owner in addition to crediting the author and publisher in your reference section.

WHEN DO YOU NEED PERMISSION?

Decisions regarding whether to merely reference quotes from published sources or whether to obtain permission of the copyright owner to use them depend on the general rules related to fair use of copyrighted work. "Fair use" is a purposefully flexible concept that cannot be specifically defined. It pertains to copying or quoting without permission of or payment to the copyright owner. Basically, such use must be reasonable and not harmful to the copyright owner.

A doctrine of fair use has existed in copyright law as a judicial interpretation for many years, but this concept is formally cited for the first time in the Copyright Act of 1976. The provisions of this act became law in January 1978.

The new law states that the fair use of a copyrighted work for purposes such as criticism, comment, news reporting, teaching (including multiple copies for classroom use), scholarship, or research is not an infringement of copyright. Four criteria are cited for determining whether a particular use can be considered fair[1].

1. The purpose and character of the use, including whether or not the use will be for profit.
2. The nature of the copyrighted work.
3. The amount or substantiality of the portion used in relation to the copyrighted work as a whole.
4. The effect of the use on the potential market for the copyrighted work.

Even when you know about and understand the concept of fair use, deciding if a particular use is fair or if permission is necessary can be difficult. One resource that can help you clarify a particular situation is *A Manual of Style,* published by the University of Chicago Press[2]. According to its guidelines, permission definitely needs to be obtained when the material used is complete in itself, such as a short story, essay, chapter from a book, article, poem, table, chart, graph, map, picture, musical composition, and so forth. Permission must also be obtained to use more than one line of a short poem still in copyright or any words to the music of a popular song. No permission is required for quoting from works in the public domain, that is, works in which the copyright has expired or never existed (such as most United States government publications). Whether an author needs to request permission to use *portions* of a published work depends on whether quoting that material falls under the doctrine of fair use of copyrighted material, (The four criteria used to determine fair use are cited in the preceding paragraph.) In determining fair use, *A Manual of Style* states that "if the quoted passage is from a published work in prose and not an entity of any sort within a larger work, and its use does not detract from the value of the original, the author should probably *not* ask permission to use it regardless of length"[3].

Figure 7.   An Example of a Permissions Request.

I. Screen
Editor
The T–Rific Publishing Company
New York, NY 10010

Dear Ms. Screen:

I am preparing an article for publication in the journal NURSE EDUCATOR as follows:

Tentative title/author: *"How to Teach" by Edu K. Torr*

Estimated publishing date: *March 1980*

I request your permission to include the following material, formerly published by the T–Rific Publishing Company, in my article. A Xerox copy of the article, with the areas permission is requested for highlighted, is included for your information.

Author(s) and/or Editor(s)   *Jane and John Grymm*

Title of book or periodical   *Educating Educators*

Title of selection   *"Keeping Your Students Awake"*   Copyright date   *1952*

from page   *123,*   line   *5,*   beginning with the words   *"Once upon a time . . .*

to page   *124,*   line   *9,*   ending with the words   *. . . happily ever after."*

Figure #_____ on page _____, Table #_____ on page _____

Please indicate agreement by signing and returning the enclosed copy of this letter. If permission from anyone else is necessary, please supply their name and address below

_____

_____

_____

Thank you for your assistance.

Edu K. Torr, R.N., Ph.D.   Old Town University
Associate Professor   Boston, MA 02171

_____   _____
(name)   (return address)

Agreed to and accepted:

by _____   _____   _____

    signature   title   date

Credit and/or Copyright Notice as you wish it to appear

Although neither the copyright act nor court decisions define fair use in terms of length of material quoted, many publishers do so. One publisher may say that not more than 150 words from an article may be quoted without permission, whereas another may set an upper limit of 500 or 1,000 words. A journal's manuscript guidelines may state the upper limit length of a quote that can be used without permission, or you can ask the editor whether the publishing company has set such a limit. Remember, however, that these rules do not have any validity outside the publishing house walls. Courts decide what is fair use, not publishers. The rules exist to give an overworked permissions department a yardstick for making decisions regarding whether proposed use of a quotation is all right, as well as, perhaps, to discourage writers from using published work unscrupulously[4].

Under the new copyright law *unpublished* material is automatically protected by copyright beginning at the time the work is created if the work has been deposited with the Library of Congress. When using such material, you need to seek permission from the author or the author's heirs[5].

HOW TO REQUEST PERMISSION

When requesting permission, send the publisher a letter that points out what published material you wish to use, identifying it by title, author, date of publication, page, and selection. State where you intend to publish it and in what context. Include a copy of your article, highlighting the material you are requesting permission for. Ask if it is also necessary to obtain the author's permission and whether the publisher has any particular preference for how the credit line should read. (See figure 7 for an example of a form letter requesting permission to quote from another source.)

ETHICAL CONSIDERATIONS

In addition to referencing accurately and getting appropriate permission to use copyrighted materials, authors need to be aware of the ethical standards that govern material that is not copyrighted but was developed by someone else. It is *not* ethical to write up content from a speech or workshop presented by another person as if that material were your own. You *can* write it, but you have to give credit to the creator.

NOTES

1. Lieb, C. H., *New Copyright Law: Overview* (New York: Association of American Publisher, 1976), p. 4.
2. *A Manual of Style,* 12th ed. (Chicago: University of Chicago Press, 1969), p. 92.
3. Ibid., p. 93.
4. Ibid., p. 93.
5. Mullins, C. J., *A Guide to Writing and Publishing in the Social and Behavioral Sciences* (New York: John Wiley and Sons, 1977), p. 30.

Chapter 8
Submit It for Publication

Sending your manuscript to the publisher requires more than a trip to the post office. You need to know certain vital statistics, such as how many copies to send and whether to double- or triple-space the typing. Always check the journal's manuscript guidelines for specific information. However, since many requirements are consistent from journal to journal, this chapter provides some general advice regarding manuscript submission.

First of all, editors want typed manuscripts with double- or triple-spacing and large margins on all sides. They often ask for two or three copies of an article to avoid having to make copies for review or editing.

With the manuscript, send a cover letter that refers to both article and journal by name. Some publishing companies have more than one journal, and you want your manuscript to land on the right desk. Also refer by date and topic to any previous correspondence between you and the editors regarding this manuscript. Editors can then retrieve the correspondence readily, an act that may have a positive effect on their decision. For example, such a letter may remind an editor that he/she encouraged the writing of this manuscript several weeks earlier. It's harder to turn down a solicited article. Not impossible or even unusual, but harder. Since editors respond to dozens of queries every week, they may not remember you without some memory jogging. In addition, be sure the cover letter carries your mailing address and telephone number.

Along with the manuscript and cover letter, include letters of permission for any materials used in the manuscript that are owned by other authors, publishers, or organizations. (See chapter seven to find out when and how to obtain permissions.)

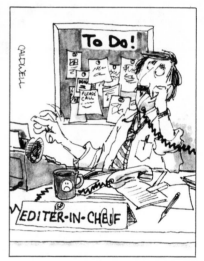

Many journals also require a short biographic sketch of the author and an abstract of the article. The manuscript guidelines will give necessary details regarding these items. The guidelines should also give the name of the editor to whom you should send the article. If not, refer to the advice in chapter three.

THE REVIEW PROCESS

After you mail the article, the long wait begins. Although the editorial process often seems too long, it may actually be proceeding as efficiently as possible. Perhaps knowing what happens during those weeks or months of waiting will be helpful.

When a publishing company receives a manuscript, a secretary usually mails an acknowledgment to the author. This form letter or postcard states that the manuscript has been received and may give some information about the next step in the process—the editor's initial review. Based on the editor's review, the article can be sent for peer review, returned for revision, accepted, or rejected. You usually hear the results of this initial review two to four weeks after the manuscript is acknowledged.

Peer Review: The Referee Process

Many professional journals are refereed; that is, experts in the field who are based outside the editorial offices review articles that have passed an initial editorial screening. The reviews heavily influence subsequent acceptance, rejection, or requests for revision. Usually two to four referees review a manuscript, providing the editor with insight regarding the content's significance, currency, and usefulness to the readership. (See "The Referee Process" in Appendix II for more information regarding refereeing.) Reviewers' advice regarding what is *not* new or useful is equally valuable. They may point out incorrect or obsolete content or poor research design. An author's revision or expansion of a manuscript based on reviewers' and editors' suggestions can make the difference between a mediocre article and one that is an important contribution to the literature.

The peer review process, coupled with professional judgment, enables editors to make informed decisions and thus develop useful content. At some journals several editors review articles, and final decisions are made at an editorial meeting where peer and editorial reviews are weighed. In addition to looking at the significance, currency, and accuracy of the content, the editors assess how clear the writing is and how the content fits into the editorial balance of future issues. After considering all these factors, the editor decides whether to accept, reject, or ask for revision of the article.

Usually the editorial process, including the time editors need to "review the reviews" and reach a decision, takes two to three months. However reviewers and editors often travel a great deal or are faced with unexpected situations that may delay the process.

Back for Revision

If your article falls into the "back for revision" category, the editor returns it requesting revision based on editorial and/or peer review suggestions. Requests for revision most often ask you to: (1) include further information deemed vital to full development of the topic; (2) clarify information presented; (3) reorganize the content. If the reviews were generally positive, editors may tell you that the manuscript will very likely be accepted following adequate revision. If you agree that the requested revision will improve the article, write immediately and tell the editors when to expect it. Let them know that it will be a superb revision which will deal competently and creatively with the issues raised. Knowing your manuscript will arrive by a certain date may prevent an editor from accepting another article on the same topic during the revision period.

What if you disagree with the suggestions for revision? Perhaps a referee misinterprets an analysis you made or the editor asks you to clarify a concept that you know the readership is already familiar with. Write back at once and clearly indicate your reservations regarding revising your manuscript according to the suggestions received. If you feel certain you are right, don't be afraid of decreasing your chances for acceptance. It's *your* manuscript and you don't want to publish anything under your name unless you fully agree with the content. Editors welcome all input that contributes to the development of accurate, useful content. The editor will probably discuss your response with the referees and may have one or two more experts in the field review the manuscript and comment on the problem area. Armed with fresh advice, the editor can then assess the situation and try to reach agreement with you regarding presentation of the information under question.

Rejection

Your first rejection will be painful—everyone's is. But as you continue a professional career that includes an average amount of writing, you'll find that some articles will be rejected while others are accepted. Gradually your ego will suffer less over the rejections. You'll probably even develop specific defenses to cope with the rejections such as the one Snoopy demonstrates in figure 8. Remember that receiving one or two rejections doesn't mean your article won't ever be published. It's possible that several journals might reject it before you find the one it's focused correctly for (see chapter two). Or the editors and/or reviewers' comments may help you revise it so its chances for acceptance are greater. Some insight into the process leading up to rejection may be helpful.

If your manuscript is rejected outright (without being sent for peer review), the rejection often comes as a form letter pointing out that

Figure 8.   Coping with Rejection.

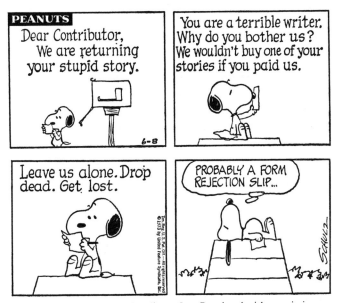

© 1973 United Feature Syndicate, Inc. Reprinted with permission.

the article "does not meet our editorial needs" or a similarly vague statement. Editors do not usually have time to give each author feedback regarding rejections that take place prior to peer review.

Such initial rejections usually occur for one or more of three reasons:

1. Poor organization and unclear writing. The editor feels it would take too much editorial time to make this manuscript publishable, even if the topic is a good one.
2. Similar material has been published recently or is awaiting publication.

3. The content is not focused for the journal's readers. (See chapter two, for more information regarding focus.)

Your article may pass the editor's initial screening but be rejected following peer review. In this case the editor should give you a more individualized report with a concrete reason or two for rejection. Authors rejected at this stage often receive a general statement regarding the reasons for rejection along with anonymous copies of the advisers' reviews to provide additional feedback.

Acceptance

If you apply what you learn from this book, and if you're persistent, sometime, someplace, you may receive that "We are pleased to inform you" letter. As soon as your initial celebrating subsides, respond to the acceptance letter. You will have a copyright agreement to fill out and the editor may need an abstract, biographical material, or other items. Letters of acceptance sometimes indicate when the editors expect copy editing to be completed and may even give an approximate publication date.

CONTACTING THE EDITOR

At various points in the editorial process you will need to communicate with the editor. For example, most editors acknowledge manuscripts immediately, but not all do. If you don't receive an acknowledgment within a month of submitting your manuscript, write the editor a brief, friendly note inquiring about its status.

A notice stating that a manuscript has been sent for peer review may indicate when you can expect to hear about the review's results. Let two or three weeks longer than the time limit given go by before writing. If no time limit is given, allow three months for peer review. In general, write to editors rather than call them. Telephone calls interrupt their work and they can't help you until your file is pulled. You may end up with a good-sized long distance telephone bill before anyone can give you specific information regarding your situation.

Unless an editor suggests you call, write first giving the specifics of the problem and ask the editor to call or write as soon as possible. Provide a telephone number and a time when you can be reached as well as your current address.

Acceptance of your article is only the beginning. Now it moves through another process, one that ends with it finally in print.

Chapter 9

From Acceptance to Publication: The Publishing Process

Your manuscript passes under many pens before it appears between the pages of a journal. At most publishing houses you can expect the following processes to occur.

COPY EDITING

The letter of acceptance usually indicates that the manuscript will go to copy editing shortly. (Most journals begin copy editing an article soon after its acceptance; a few wait until a few months before they plan to publish it.)

What to Expect

"Copy editing" can mean anything from inserting commas to substantial rewriting. When authors' state their message well, according to the principles of clear writing cited in chapter five, editing will usually be light. (Publishers call such editing, which focuses on details of style such as punctuation or agreement of subject and verb, *mechanical* editing.)

However, professionals and academics are noted for their wordiness and propensity to "gobbledygook," and an overwritten or cloudy manuscript will set editors to cutting, slashing, and sometimes rewriting. Editors call such a process *substantive* editing. The editor may get rid of unnecessary words, substitute simpler words for complex ones, put sentences in active voice, place important points at the ends of sentences, and break up long paragraphs. At times an editor will reorganize a manuscript—also in the interests of clarity — by that extremely sophisticated technique known as "cutting and pasting." Remember that throughout the editing process, no matter how they seem to cut and slash at your work, good copy editors subscribe to the ethic of preserving an author's meaning at all cost and an author's style as far as possible. When such a copy editor finishes with your manuscript it may not look like the same one you submitted, but when you read it your meaning should ring true. And now it's not just meaningful to you; others will also be able to comprehend it.

Reaction to Editing

Most journals will tell you on acceptance that you will be sent the copy-edited manuscript for review of the editing before publication. Figure 9, an example of mechanical editing, will help you understand the various copy editing marks. If the editors don't mention sending the copy-edited manuscript for review when they accept your article, ask them about it when you respond to the acceptance letter. Authors should always review an edited manuscript prior to publication, for there may be editorial changes that do change meaning or are otherwise unacceptable. The post copy-editing period is the time to make any changes. Typesetting follows, and once the type is set it becomes very expensive to change even a few words.

When reviewing the edited manuscript, enter all definite changes neatly and legibly on the manuscript, using a different color ink from the copy editor's. If you are merely suggesting changes, enter them in pencil or on a separate sheet of paper. Remember that the typesetter will have to read your insertions, for it's unlikely that any part of the manuscript will be retyped. List the pages and paragraphs where you have made changes on a separate sheet of paper, and send this to the editor along with the edited manuscript.

Figure 9. Example of an Edited Manuscript.

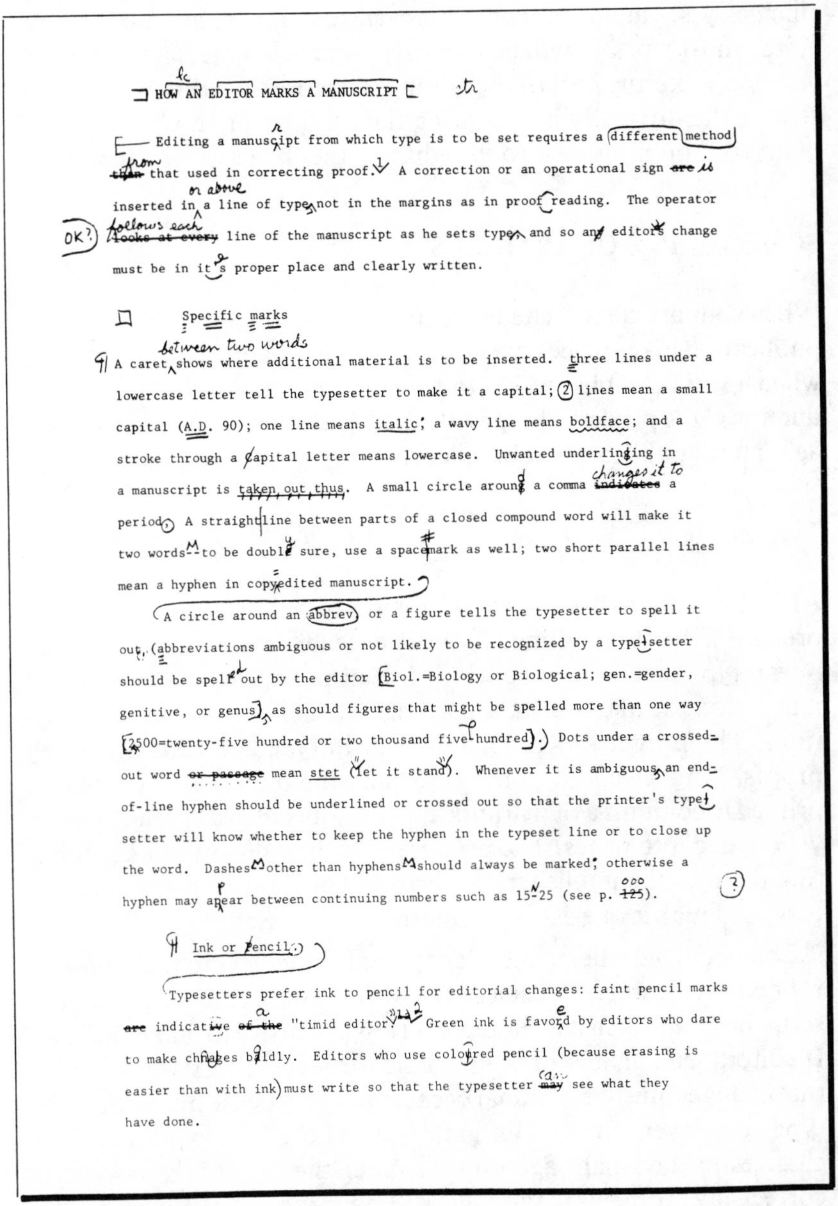

HOW AN EDITOR MARKS A MANUSCRIPT

Editing a manuscipt from which type is to be set requires a different method than that used in correcting proof. A correction or an operational sign are inserted in a line of type, not in the margins as in proof reading. The operator looks at every line of the manuscript as he sets type, and so any editors change must be in it's proper place and clearly written.

Specific marks

A caret shows where additional material is to be inserted. three lines under a lowercase letter tell the typesetter to make it a capital; 2 lines mean a small capital (A.D. 90); one line means italic; a wavy line means boldface; and a stroke through a capital letter means lowercase. Unwanted underlinging in a manuscript is taken out thus. A small circle aroung a comma indicates a period. A straight line between parts of a closed compound word will make it two words--to be double sure, use a spacemark as well; two short parallel lines mean a hyphen in copyedited manuscript.

A circle around an abbrev or a figure tells the typesetter to spell it out, (abbreviations ambiguous or not likely to be recognized by a typesetter should be spelt out by the editor (Biol.=Biology or Biological; gen.=gender, genitive, or genus), as should figures that might be spelled more than one way (2500=twenty-five hundred or two thousand five hundred).) Dots under a crossed-out word or passage mean stet (let it stand). Whenever it is ambiguous, an end-of-line hyphen should be underlined or crossed out so that the printer's type-setter will know whether to keep the hyphen in the typeset line or to close up the word. Dashes--other than hyphens--should always be marked; otherwise a hyphen may apear between continuing numbers such as 15-25 (see p. 125).

Ink or Pencil.

Typesetters prefer ink to pencil for editorial changes: faint pencil marks are indicative of the "timid editor." Green ink is favord by editors who dare to make chnages boldly. Editors who use colored pencil (because erasing is easier than with ink) must write so that the typesetter may see what they have done.

From *A Manual of Style.* Chicago: The University of Chicago Press, 1969, p. 41. Reprinted with permission.

When you return the manuscript, send a cover letter indicating your acceptance of the editing or pointing out any copy-editing changes you cannot accept. However, remember that author and editor must work together to clarify an article's message. Thus, if you don't like any part of the editing, do more than disagree. Try to resolve the difficulty by rewriting the problem area. Carefully explain your point of view to the editor, either by letter or telephone.

SCHEDULING OF ARTICLES

When your article is "scheduled" (about two to three months before publication takes place), you usually receive a notice stating exactly when it will be published. At this point, your manuscript is "in production," the process of typesetting and printing. You may not see it again until publication takes place.

Typesetting

After the author has approved a copy-edited manuscript, editors prepare it for typesetting. Type size, leading (space between the lines), type face, and type width for all parts are determined and marked on the manuscript according to the printer's type specifications. The printer sets the manuscript in type and runs off galley proofs, long sheets of paper on which the manuscript content is printed in columns as it will appear in the journal, except that it is not yet divided into pages. The printer reads the galleys before submitting them to the publisher, corrects any obvious typographical errors, and makes queries in the margin, if necessary.

Some journal editors submit copies of the galleys to their authors for review. However, most let authors review the copy-edited manuscript instead, when it is simpler and less expensive to make changes. If editors send galleys of your article for review, they will stipulate that changes must be minimal because of the expense of resetting the type. However, changes in galley prints are less expensive than changes in the final page proofs. After the printer resets type to correct any problems in the galleys, the appropriate editorial or production staff person "lays out" the article, spacing it as it will appear in the journal. The printer then runs off page proofs, often known as "blues" because they are printed on blue paper. Editors scrutinize the page proofs in one final check before sending the articles and other content for a specific issue off for actual printing.

Printing

Writers don't really need to know the details of typesetting and printing, but a passing familiarity with the different processes and terms may help them feel more comfortable in dealing with publishers. Basically, four types of printing processes exist: letterpress, offset, gravure, and silkscreen.

Letterpress printing consists of *mechanical* reproduction where impressions are made on paper from a metal plate with inked raised surfaces. Thus, each letter is essentially cast in metal and pressed against paper. Letterpress printing is sometimes referred to as the "hot type" method. It used to be the major means of printing all books, newspapers, and magazines, but now the more flexible offset printing process is often used.

Offset printing is done by chemical means. The process is based on the principle that water and grease won't mix. A photographic image of each page is made and transferred to a metal plate set on a roller where it is treated so that the nonprinted area will repel ink. The inked image is then transferred to a rubber blanket roller and from the blanket to paper. Today, most magazines use offset rather than letterpress because of its greater flexibility and lower cost.

Gravure is a photomechanical printing process in which printing is done from an engraved copper cylinder. The inked areas (letters, pictures, and so on) are depressed (etched in), not raised as in letterpress. It is used for printing cartons, vinyl floor coverings, and postage stamps.

Silkscreen printing is done by treating cloth with an impermeable coating except where the color is to be forced through onto paper. It is primarily used for such items as art prints, posters, and wallpaper and for printing on textiles, leather, glass, and wood.

FINALLY PUBLISHED

Following the publication of an article, authors often receive complimentary copies of the journal it appears in and/or a number of reprints. If the publishing company does not provide free reprints, it may sell them to authors at a reduced price. Some journals pay authors an honorarium.

NOTES

1. *A Manual of Style,* 12th ed. (Chicago: University of Chicago Press, 1969).

BIBLIOGRAPHY
Barnhart, C.L., *The American College Dictionary. New York: Random House, 1961.*
A Manual of Style, 12th ed. Chicago: University of Chicago Press, 1969. Moyes, N. B., and White, D. M., *Journalism in the Mass Media.* Lexington, Mass.: Ginn and Co., 1974.
Nicholson, M., *A Practical Style Guide for Authors and Editors.* New York: Holt, Reinhart and Winston, 1967.
Pocket Pal: *A Graphic Arts Production Handbook,* 11th ed. New York: International Paper Co., 1974.

Chapter 10
Copyright Law

What do authors need to know about copyright law? They should understand the concept of copyright and their rights, as authors, regarding the material they create. In addition, they need to be able to apply this understanding to a specific publishing situation and make an informed decision regarding whether to retain their rights to articles or other content, or to transfer full or partial ownership of copyright to their publishers. This chapter defines copyright and provides information that will help authors make such decisions.

DEFINITION

Copyright: The exclusive right granted by law for a certain number of years, to make and dispose of copies of, and otherwise to control, a literary, musical or artistic work[1].

The copyright holder has the exclusive right to control the printing publication, and other uses of a work for a specified period of time. Under the Copyright Act of 1976, which took effect in January 1978, this period consists of the author's lifetime plus fifty years.

The copyright law was conceived to encourage the development and distribution of works of authorship. It seeks to accomplish this objective by giving authors certain exclusive rights to their work, including the right to authorize others to exercise those rights. If such protection were absent, unauthorized reproduction and distribution would be so easily accomplished that the quantity and diversity of creative activity would decrease[2].

AUTHOR'S RIGHTS

The most important revision incorporated in the Copyright Act of 1976, which amends the Copyright Act of 1909, is the change in copyright ownership. Publishers can no longer assume ownership of copyright to material published in their magazines unless they specifically obtain those rights from authors[3].

Under the new law, the author of an original work is the initial owner of the copyright in that work and owns the exclusive rights of copyright: reproduction, preparation of derivative works, public distribution, public performance, and public display. In a joint work, that is, one prepared by two or more authors, the authors are co-owners of copyright.

In collective works such as anthologies, periodicals, and encyclopedias, copyright for the work as a whole is separate from copyright for each individual contribution. The owner of copyright in the work as a whole is not automatically the owner of copyright for each contribution. Under the old law that was sometimes the case. Under the new law, a specific rule applies. In the absence of an express transfer of the copyright or of any rights under it, the owner of copyright in the collective work has acquired only the privilege of reproducing and distributing the contribution as part of: (1) that particular collective work; (2) any revision of that collective work; (3) any later collective work in the same series (the same magazine)[4].

TRANSFER OF COPYRIGHT OWNERSHIP

Thus, from the time of a work's creation, the author owns all rights to it unless those rights or any subdivision of them are transferred by a written instrument signed by the owner[5].

What does all of this mean for the author whose article is accepted for publication in a professional journal?

Under the old copyright law, authors usually signed a statement verifying that the material accepted for publication was not being considered for publication elsewhere. Upon publication the publisher assumed copyright ownership of part or all of the rights to the article. If the publisher held "all rights" it meant that the author forfeited the right to use the material in the same form elsewhere. More often publishers assumed "first serial rights" giving the periodical the right to be the first to publish the work. All other rights remained with the author. However, the publisher held these rights as trustee of the author and assigned them to him only upon written request.

Whether publishers assumed all rights or first serial rights was usually part of their publishing policy. Often authors didn't know what rights publishers had to their articles unless they specifically requested information. Many pre-1978 guide books for free-lance writers suggest that writers type "first serial rights only" at the top of their manuscripts when submitting them. If a manuscript bearing that statement was accepted, the publisher would be assuming only first serial rights, the right to publish the article once. However, since the publisher held other rights as trustee of the author, he/she could grant permission to other parties to reprint the article and make other decisions regarding it.

Under the new law, if publishers wish to have the capability of producing or granting permission to others to produce reprints, books, or motion pictures based on articles, stories, or poems they publish, they must ask the author to transfer the copyright to them by a legal, written agreement. Thus, shortly after the Copyright Act of 1976 was passed, publishing houses began drawing up letters, often called copyright transfer agreements or publishing agreements, for authors' signatures. Such a letter effects transfer of full or partial copyright to the publisher.

Authors may wish to separate the rights they keep and those they transfer to their publishers. For example, if an author wishes to retain book rights, a transfer agreement can stipulate that a publishing company owns "exclusive worldwide magazine rights including the right to reprint in hard copy or microfilm, excerpt rights, foreign language rights, data base publishing rights, and the right to grant the foregoing to third parties." The letter would also state, "We understand you retain the book rights."

Thus, authors retain all rights to their work unless they sign a written agreement to transfer them. Authors may rightfully be confused about whether to sign a copyright transfer agreement giving the publisher all rights or work out retention of specific rights. Many publishers will encourage authors to transfer full copyright to the publishing company even in cases where they don't expect to profit from owning the rights because full ownership simplifies future permissions processes for them. Some publishers won't accept articles unless authors transfer full copyright to them.

HOW DOES OWNING AN ARTICLE BENEFIT A PUBLISHER?

In addition to simplifying administration of permissions, full copyright ownership entitles the publisher to the following:

1. Royalties on microfilm editions of the journal
2. Profits on the sale of reprints
3. Profits should the article be included in an anthology the publisher develops following its publication in the journal. If a publishing company owns the copyright to an article, it is not obliged to even inform the author of such future use, although most publishers do so as a matter of courtesy.
4. The right to generate videotapes, filmstrips, films, and audio cassettes. For example, suppose an article is presented in script form. By hiring professionals to "read" it, audio cassettes with high potential sales could be produced.
5. Control of all subsequent reprinting. Most publishers would probably agree to any future use that authors want to make of their own articles, but they are not obliged to do so. For instance, if an author wanted to publish an article that had appeared in one publisher's journal in an anthology to be published by another company, the first company has the right to refuse if it owns the copyright.

SHOULD YOU TRANSFER FULL COPYRIGHT OWNERSHIP?

Whether you should transfer copyright depends on the journal and the article. You need to assess the article's profit-making potential. Most articles published in scholarly or professional journals do not have potential for large profit through their future use, and so publishers are not asking for anything valuable when they ask for complete copyright ownership. They are primarily trying to simplify future permissions processes. In such cases authors probably save themselves time and money in administering permissions requests if they transfer copyright ownership to the publisher.

In determining whether your material has profit-making potential through its future use, you should ask yourself whether an article could become a videotape, filmstrip, film, audio cassette, or a valuable addition to an anthology. If one or more of these seems likely, it would be in your best interest to grant the publisher only the right to publish the article once in the journal. Then if that publisher developed plans for other uses of the materials, you would be asked to renegotiate terms for each use and would share in the profits.

As authors become increasingly accustomed to dealing with the new copyright law, they will probably find that some of their articles are worth the time and negotiation necessary to retain certain rights. Others will not have the reuse potential to be worth the effort. In all cases, basic understanding of current copyright law will help authors make informed, individual decisions in their best interests.

NOTES

1. *The American College Dictionary* (New York: Random House, 1961), p. 268.
2. Johnston, D. F., *The Copyright Handbook* (New York: R. R. Bowker Co., 1978), p. xiii.
3. Love, B., Coping with copyright: revised laws give authors new clout. *Folio* 7(2):18.
4. Johnston, D. F., *The Copyright Handbook* (New York: R. R. Bowker Co., 1978), pp. 46-47.
5. The new copyright law, some observations. *The Huenefeld Report,* August 22, 1977, p. 2.

Appendix I

Journals that Offer Publishing Opportunities for Nurses

Information follows regarding 74 journals in which nurses might publish. An asterisk (*) indicates journals that responded to a 1979 request to update information originally published in 1977 (McCloskey, J.C. Publishing opportunities for nurses: a comparison of 65 journals. *Nurse Educator,* 2 (4):4–12.) as well as new journals surveyed for the first time in 1979. In addition to updating the 1977 information, the 1979 survey asked journal editors to indicate each journal's referee status. The question on referee status was worded: "Is your journal refereed? (Do experts in a particular field, such as nursing, review manuscripts and provide input to editorial decisions?)"

If no asterisk appears, the journal did not respond to the request to update content published in 1977. Thus the information provided was obtained prior to the 1977 publication date and no information regarding referee status is offered.

General Nursing

A.J.N. (American Journal of Nursing)
555 West 57th Street
New York, NY 10019

Circulation:	350,000
Organizational association:	American Nurses' Association
Yearly frequency:	12x
Average article length:	1,500–2,500 words
Number of copies to submit (including original):	2
Author payment:	$20/page
Reprints:	100 free for exclusively prepared material
Time for editorial decision:	several weeks
Time for publication of accepted manuscript:	2–18 months
Solicited articles published per year:	35 percent
Unsolicited articles published per year:	65 percent
Acceptance rate for unsolicited articles:	10 percent
Refereed?	large staff of nurse editors representing various fields of nursing, supplemented by use of consultants when necessary in editors' judgment. This parallels other journals' use of boards

*Nursing
132 Welsh Road
Horsham, PA 19044

Circulation:	500,000
Circulation:	none
Yearly frequency:	12x
Average article length:	1,500–3,000 words
Number of copies to submit (including original):	2
Author payment:	$100–$350 per article
Reprints:	1 journal copy free
Time for editorial decision:	6–8 weeks
Time for publication of accepted manuscript:	6–12 months
Solicited articles published per year:	most
Unsolicited articles published per year:	some
Acceptance rate for unsolicited articles:	5–10 percent
Refereed?	yes

*Nursing and Health Care
265 Post Road West
Westport, CT 06880

Circulation:	25,000
Organizational association:	National League for Nursing
Yearly frequency:	10 times yearly, September through June
Average article length:	3,600 to 4,200 words
Number of copies to submit (including original):	original and two copies
Author payment:	none
Reprints:	100
Time for editorial decision:	2–3 months
Time for publication of accepted manuscript:	2–18 months*
Solicited articles published per year:	50 percent*
Unsolicited articles published per year:	none yet
Acceptance rate for unsolicited articles:	50 percent*
Refereed?	yes

*these are projected figures as the inaugural issue was published in August, 1980

*The Nursing Clinics of North America
W. Washington Square
Philadelphia, PA 19105

Circulation:	30,000
Organizational association:	none
Yearly frequency:	4x
Average article length:	3,600 words
Number of copies to submit (including original):	1
Author payment:	$100 to guest editor
Reprints:	100 free and one journal
Time for editorial decision:	not applicable, see below
Time for publication of accepted manuscript:	6 months–1 year
Solicited articles published per year:	nearly 100 percent
Unsolicited articles published per year:	2–5
Acceptance rate for unsolicited articles:	rare
Refereed?	Not according to this definition, but our guest editors who are experts in their field select the contributors and topics for each article and review the papers received. Thus they act as "semi-referees".

RN
Medical Economics Co.
Oradell, NJ 07649

Circulation:	205,000
Organizational association:	none
Yearly frequency:	12x
Average article length:	2,000–2,500 words
Number of copies to submit (including original):	2
Author payment:	$50–200 article
Reprints:	at cost
Time for editorial decision:	2–3 weeks
Time for publication of accepted manuscript:	3 months
Solicited articles published per year:	most
Unsolicited articles published per year:	many
Acceptance rate for unsolicited articles:	10 percent

Specialty Nursing

*Advances in Nursing Science
Aspen Systems Corporation
1600 Research Blvd.
Rockville, MD 20850

Circulation:	3,019
Organizational association:	none
Yearly frequency:	quarterly
Average article length:	4,000 words
Number of copies to submit (including original):	3
Author payment:	none
Reprints:	on request for a fee
Time for editorial decision:	8 weeks
Time for publication of accepted manuscript:	6 months
Solicited articles published per year:	10
Unsolicited articles published per year:	35 (Note: Each issue is devoted entirely to one topic. A list of upcoming issue topics is available from the publisher.)
Refereed?	yes

AORN Journal
Association Operating Room Nurses, Inc.
10170 E. Mississippi Avenue
Denver, CO 80231

Circulation:	27,719
Organizational association:	Association of Operating Room Nurses
Yearly frequency:	13x
Average article length:	3,000 words
Number of copies to submit (including original):	2
Author payment:	none
Reprints:	at editor's discretion
Time for editorial decision:	1–6 months
Time for publication of accepted manuscript:	2–12 months
Solicited articles published per year:	25
Unsolicited articles published per year:	75
Acceptance rate for unsolicited articles:	60 percent

*Cardiovascular Nursing
American Heart Association
7320 Greenville Avenue
Dallas, TX 75231

Circulation: 120,000

Organizational association: American Heart Association

Yearly frequency: 6x

Average article length: 3,000 words

Number of copies to submit
(including original):   2

Author payment: none

Reprints: not supplied

Time for editorial decision: 4–6 weeks

Time for publication of
accepted manuscript: 5–6 months

Solicited articles
published per year: most

Unsolicited articles
published per year: few

Acceptance rate for
unsolicited articles: 12–20 percent

Refereed?   yes

*Heart and Lung: The Journal of Critical Care
33 W. First Street
Dayton, OH 45402

Circulation: 57,000

Organizational association: American Association of Critical
                                                     Care Nurses

Yearly frequency: 6x

Average article length: 3,750 words

Number of copies to submit
(including original):   2

Author payment: none

Reprints: at cost

Time for editorial decision: 4–6 weeks

Time for publication of
accepted manuscript: 5–6 months

Solicited articles
published per year: 10–12

Unsolicited articles
published per year: 90

Acceptance rate for
unsolicited articles: 40 percent

Refereed?   yes

Imprint
National Student Nurses' Association, Inc.
W. Columbus Circle
New York, NY 10019

Circulation:	40,000
Organizational association:	National Student Nurses' Association
Yearly frequency:	5x
Average article length:	1,500–2,000 words
Number of copies to submit (including original):	2
Author payment:	none
Reprints:	some free
Time for editorial decision:	2 months
Time for publication of accepted manuscript:	12 months
Solicited articles published per year:	1/3 of articles published
Unsolicited articles published per year:	2/3 of articles published
Acceptance rate for unsolicited articles:	50 percent
Refereed?	all copy is screened by student nurse editor

*Journal of Emergency Nursing
Emergency Department Nurses Association
666 North Lake Shore Drive, Suite 1729
Chicago, IL 60611

Circulation:	14,000
Organizational association:	Emergency Department Nurses Association
Yearly frequency:	bimonthly (6 times a year)
Average article length:	5,000 words
Number of copies to submit (including original):	3
Author payment:	none
Reprints:	authors get 3 copies of the journal
Time for editorial decision:	3 months
Time for publication of accepted manuscript:	9 months
Solicited articles published per year:	25
Unsolicited articles published per year:	50
Acceptance rate for unsolicited articles:	60 percent
Refereed?	yes; each article is reviewed by two or three emergency nurses with experience in the area covered by the manuscript

Journal of Neurosurgical Nursing
c/o: Williams and Wilkins Co.
428 E. Preston Street
Baltimore, MD 21202

Circulation:	2,000
Organizational association:	American Association of Neurosurgical Nurses
Yearly frequency:	4x
Average article length:	varies
Number of copies to submit (including original):	2
Author payment:	none
Reprints:	at cost
Time for editorial decision:	2–3months
Time for publication of accepted manuscript:	12 months
Solicited articles published per year:	
Unsolicited articles published per year:	publishes monthly manuscripts that members present at annual meetings
Acceptance rate for unsolicited articles:	

*Journal of Nurse-Midwifery
1012 14th Street, N.W.—Suite 801
Washington, D.C. 20005

Circulation: 3,900

Organizational association: American College of Nurse
                                                       Midwifes

Yearly frequency: 6x

Average article length: 2,500–5,000 words

Number of copies to submit
(including original):   2

Author payment: none

Reprints: at cost in orders of 100 or up

Time for editorial decision: 3 months

Time for publication of
accepted manuscript: 6–9 months

Solicited articles
published per year: none

Unsolicited articles
published per year: 50–60

Acceptance rate for
unsolicited articles: 50 percent

Refereed?   yes, by an editorial board
                                                       composed of certified nurse-
                                                       midwives (CNMs)

*The Journal of Nursing Administration
12 Lakeside Park
607 North Avenue
Wakefield, MA 01880

Circulation:	17,000
Organizational association:	none
Yearly frequency:	12x
Average article length:	varies
Number of copies to submit (including original):	3
Author payment:	$75/article
Reprints:	at cost
Time for editorial decision:	4–8 weeks
Time for publication of accepted manuscript:	6–10 months
Solicited articles published per year:	25
Unsolicited articles published per year:	40
Acceptance rate for unsolicited articles:	35 percent
Refereed?	partial

*Journal of Nursing Education
Charles B. Slack, Inc.
6900 Grove Road
Thorofare, NJ 08086

Circulation: 3,300

Organizational association: none

Yearly frequency: 9x

Average article length: 2,000–3,000 words

Number of copies to submit
(including original):   2

Author payment: none

Reprints: at cost

Time for editorial decision: 6 weeks

Time for publication of
accepted manuscript: 6–12 months

Solicited articles
published per year: few

Unsolicited articles
published per year: most

Acceptance rate for
unsolicited articles: 40 percent

Refereed?   yes

*JOGN (Journal of Obstetric, Gynecologic and Neonatal Nursing)
One East Wacker Drive, Suite 2700
Chicago, IL 60601

Circulation:	27,000
Organizational association:	Nurses Association of the American College of Obstetricians and Gynecologists
Yearly frequency:	6x
Average article length:	2,500–5,000 words
Number of copies to submit (including original):	2
Author payment:	none
Reprints:	at cost
Time for editorial decision:	2–4 months
Time for publication of accepted manuscript:	6–12 months
Solicited articles published per year:	5
Unsolicited articles published per year:	45
Acceptance rate for unsolicited articles:	65 percent
Refereed?	yes

Maternal Child Nursing Journal
3505 Fifth Avenue
Pittsburgh, PA 15213

Circulation: 1,000

Organizational association: graduate faculties of maternal
                                                           and pediatric nurses, University
                                                           of Pittsburgh

Yearly frequency: 4x

Average article length: 2,500–5,000 words

Number of copies to submit
(including original):   2

Author payment: none

Reprints: 100 free

Time for editorial decision: 3–6 months

Time for publication of
accepted manuscript: 3–9 months

Solicited articles
published per year: few

Unsolicited articles
published per year: most

Acceptance rate for
unsolicited articles: 75 percent

*MCN, The American Journal of Maternal Child Nursing
555 West 57th Street
New York, NY 10019

Circulation:	25,000
Organizational association:	none
Yearly frequency:	6x
Average article length:	2,500–3,250 words
Number of copies to submit (including original):	2
Author payment:	none
Reprints:	100 free
Time for editorial decision:	6 weeks
Time for publication of accepted manuscript:	up to 1 year
Solicited articles published per year:	10
Unsolicited articles published per year:	50
Acceptance rate for unsolicited articles:	25 percent

Nurse Educator
12 Lakeside Park
607 North Avenue
Wakefield, MA 01880

Circulation: 38,000

Organizational association: none

Yearly frequency: 6x

Average article length: 2,500–3,500 words

Number of copies to submit
(including original):   3

Author payment: none

Reprints: at cost

Time for editorial decision: 6–8 weeks

Time for publication of
accepted manuscript: 3–10 months

Solicited articles
published per year: 12–18

Unsolicited articles
published per year: 12–18

Acceptance rate for
unsolicited articles: 30 percent

Refereed?   partial

***The Nurse Practitioner: The American Journal
of Primary Health Care*
3845 42nd N.E.
Seattle, WA 98105**

Circulation:	6,000
Organizational association:	none, but supports nursing organizations
Yearly frequency:	bimonthly
Average article length:	8–10 double-spaced pages
Number of copies to submit (including original):	3
Author payment:	none
Reprints:	none
Time for editorial decision:	4–6 weeks
Time for publication of accepted manuscript:	depends on the content and length of material
Solicited articles published per year:	–
Unsolicited articles published per year:	approximately 50
Acceptance rate for unsolicited articles:	35 percent
Refereed?	yes; each manuscript reviewed by two members of the editorial board and by a specialist in the field of the content

*Nursing Administration Quarterly
Aspen Systems Corporation
1600 Research Blvd.
Rockville, MD 20850

Circulation:	4,439
Organizational association:	none
Yearly frequency:	quarterly
Average article length:	4,700 words
Number of copies to submit (including original):	3
Author payment:	none
Reprints:	on request for a fee
Time for editorial decision:	2 months
Time for publication of accepted manuscript:	3½ months
Solicited articles published per year:	20
Unsolicited articles published per year:	12 (Note: Each issue is devoted entirely to one topic. A list of upcoming issue topics is available from the publisher.)
Refereed?	yes

*Nursing Leadership
Charles B. Slack, Inc.
6900 Grove Road
Thorofare, NJ 08086

Circulation:	4,000
Organizational association:	none
Yearly frequency:	quarterly
Average article length:	3,000 words
Number of copies to submit (including original):	2
Author payment:	none
Reprints:	may be purchased, page count determines cost
Time for editorial decision:	6 weeks
Time for publication of accepted manuscript:	too new to judge
Solicited articles published per year:	too new to judge
Unsolicited articles published per year:	too new to judge
Acceptance rate for unsolicited articles:	too new to judge
Refereed?	yes

*Nursing Outlook
555 West 57th Street
New York, NY 10019

Circulation:	28,000
Organizational association:	none
Yearly frequency:	12x
Average article length:	2,000–4,000 words
Number of copies to submit (including original):	2
Author payment:	none
Reprints:	100 free
Time for editorial decision:	6–8 weeks
Time for publication of accepted manuscript:	4–6 months
Solicited articles published per year:	10–15
Unsolicited articles published per year:	85
Acceptance rate for unsolicited articles:	10 percent
Refereed?	for some, but not all, articles

Nursing Research
University of Pennsylvania School of Nursing
420 Service Drive
Philadelphia, PA 19104

Circulation:	8,000
Organizational association:	American Nurses' Association
Yearly frequency:	6x
Average article length:	3,500 words
Number of copies to submit (including original):	4
Author payment:	none
Reprints:	at cost
Time for editorial decision:	3 months
Time for publication of accepted manuscript:	8–12 months
Solicited articles published per year:	few
Unsolicited articles published per year:	60
Acceptance rate for unsolicited articles:	20 percent
Refereed?	yes

*Occupational Health Nursing
Charles B. Slack, Inc.
6900 Grove Road
Thorofare, NJ 08086

Circulation:	12,000
Organizational association:	American Association of Industrial Nurses, Inc.
Yearly frequency:	12x
Average article length:	3,000 words
Number of copies to submit (including original):	2
Author payment:	none
Reprints:	at cost
Time for editorial decision:	1 month
Time for publication of accepted manuscript:	3 months
Solicited articles published per year:	30
Unsolicited articles published per year:	20
Acceptance rate for unsolicited articles:	50 percent
Refereed?	yes

*Research in Nursing and Health
c/o Harriet H. Werley, Ph.D.
School of Nursing
University of Missouri—Columbia
Columbia, MO 65212

Circulation: 1,000

Organizational association: none

Yearly frequency: quarterly

Average article length: 6,000 words

Number of copies to submit
(including original):   4

Author payment: none

Reprints: 100 free reprints to first author

Time for editorial decision: 2 months

Time for publication of
accepted manuscript: 3 months

Solicited articles
published per year: 0

Unsolicited articles
published per year: 90

Acceptance rate for
unsolicited articles: 22 percent

Refereed?   yes

*Supervisor Nurse
3734 Glenway Avenue
Cincinnati, OH 45205

Circulation:	80,000
Organizational association:	none
Yearly frequency:	12x
Average article length:	2.000–4,000 words
Number of copies to submit (including original):	2
Author payment:	$50
Reprints:	at cost
Time for editorial decision:	2–8 weeks
Time for publication of accepted manuscript:	12–18 months
Solicited articles published per year:	10 percent
Unsolicited articles published per year:	90 percent
Acceptance rate for unsolicited articles:	40 percent
Refereed?	no

Topics in Clinical Nursing
Aspen Systems Corporation
1600 Research Blvd.
Rockville, MD 20850

Circulation:	5,094
Organizational association:	none
Yearly frequency:	quarterly
Average article length:	4,500 words
Number of copies to submit (including original):	2
Author payment:	none
Reprints:	on request for a fee
Time for editorial decision:	3–9 months
Time for publication of accepted manuscript:	3–9 months
Solicited articles published per year:	32
Unsolicited articles published per year:	4 (Note: Each issue is devoted entirely to one topic. A list of upcoming topics is available from the publisher.)
Refereed?	yes

Foreign Nursing

*Australian Nurses Journal
P.O. Box 197
Port Adelaide, South Australia 5015
Australia

Circulation:	being updated (was 18,000 in 1977)
Organizational association:	no response
Yearly frequency:	11x
Average article length:	2,000–3,000 words
Number of copies to submit (including original):	1
Author payment:	$50
Reprints:	at cost
Time for editorial decision:	no response
Time for publication of accepted manuscript:	nearest issue
Solicited articles published per year:	no response
Unsolicited articles published per year:	no response
Acceptance rate for unsolicited articles:	any worthwhile paper
Refereed?	no

Australian Nurses' Journal
Royal Australian Nursing Federation
33 Queens Road–Suite 18
Melbourne, Vic. 3004, Australia

Circulation:	14,000
Organizational association:	Royal Australian Nursing Federation
Yearly frequency:	12x
Average article length:	2,000–2,500 words
Number of copies to submit (including original):	1
Author payment:	variable
Reprints:	at cost
Time for editorial decision:	no response
Time for publication of accepted manuscript:	2–3 months
Solicited articles published per year:	20
Unsolicited articles published per year:	45
Acceptance rate for unsolicited articles:	40 percent

*Canada's Mental Health (Saute Mentale au Canada)
Health Services Directorate
Jeanne Mauce, 324
Tienney's Pasture
Ottawa, Ont. K1A 1B4
Canada

Circulation:	30,000
Organizational association:	Minister of National Health & Welfare
Yearly frequency:	4x
Average article length:	no response
Number of copies to submit (including original):	2
Author payment:	none
Reprints:	7 journal copies free
Time for editorial decision:	3–6 months
Time for publication of accepted manuscript:	3–6 months
Solicited articles published per year:	no response
Unsolicited articles published per year:	most
Acceptance rate for unsolicited articles:	no response
Refereed?	yes

Canadian Journal of Public Health
55 Parkdale Avenue
Ottawa, Ont. K1Y 1ES, Canada

Circulation: 5,000

Organizational association: Canadian Public Health
                                    Association

Yearly frequency: 6x

Average article length: 1,000–1,500 words

Number of copies to submit
(including original):   2

Author payment: none

Reprints: at cost

Time for editorial decision: varies

Time for publication of
accepted manuscript: 18 months

Solicited articles
published per year: no response

Unsolicited articles
published per year: 50

Acceptance rate for
unsolicited articles: 90 percent

*The Canadian Nurse
Canadian Nurses Association
Association Des Infirmieres Et
50 The Driveway
Ottawa, Canada K2P 1E2

Circulation:	97,000
Organizational association:	Canadian Nurses Association
Yearly frequency:	11x
Average article length:	1,000–2,500 words
Number of copies to submit (including original):	2
Author payment:	honorarium
Reprints:	3 journal copies free
Time for editorial decision:	4–6 weeks
Time for publication of accepted manuscript:	varies
Solicited articles published per year:	some
Unsolicited articles published per year:	most
Acceptance rate for unsolicited articles:	25 percent
Refereed?	as necessary

The Chest, Heart and Stroke Journal
The Chest, Heart and Stroke Association
Tavistock House
Tavistock Square, London WC1H9JE
England

Circulation:	6,000
Organizational association:	The Chest, Heart and Stroke Association
Yearly frequency:	4x
Average article length:	2,500 words
Number of copies to submit (including original):	2
Author payment:	by negotiation
Reprints:	at cost
Time for editorial decision:	no response
Time for publication of accepted manuscript:	3–6 months
Solicited articles published per year:	most
Unsolicited articles published per year:	very few
Acceptance rate for unsolicited articles:	very few

*CURATIONIS
South African Nursing Association
Private Bag X105
Pretoria 0001
South Africa

Circulation:	4,000
Organizational association:	none
Yearly frequency:	quarterly publication
Average article length:	1,500–5,000 words
Number of copies to submit (including original):	2
Author payment:	none
Reprints:	quotes for reprints
Time for editorial decision:	depends on nature of article
Time for publication of accepted manuscript:	can be fairly lengthy
Solicited articles published per year:	majority
Unsolicited articles published per year:	few
Acceptance rate for unsolicited articles:	no response

Hong Kong Nursing Journal
Post Office Box 3868
Sheung Wan, Hong Kong

Circulation:	4,000
Organizational association:	Hong Kong Nurses Association
Yearly frequency:	2x
Average article length:	3,000 words
Number of copies to submit (including original):	2
Author payment:	no response
Reprints:	10–20 free
Time for editorial decision:	no response
Time for publication of accepted manuscript:	1 month
Solicited articles published per year:	most
Unsolicited articles published per year:	few
Acceptance rate for unsolicited articles:	no response

***India Christian Nurse*
Christian Nurses League
Christian Medical Association of India
P.O. Box 24, Christian Council Lodge
Nagpue 440001 Mah., India

Circulation:	1,500
Organizational association:	none
Yearly frequency:	6x
Average article length:	300–500 words
Number of copies to submit (including original):	2
Author payment:	none
Reprints:	a few journal copies free
Time for editorial decision:	1 month
Time for publication of accepted manuscript:	2 months
Solicited articles published per year:	2
Unsolicited articles published per year:	no response
Acceptance rate for unsolicited articles:	no response
Refereed?	on occasion

International Council of Nurses
P.O. Box 42
CH-1211 Geneva 20 Switzerland

Circulation:	4,000
Organizational association:	International Council of Nurses
Yearly frequency:	6x
Average article length:	1,500–3,000 words
Number of copies to submit (including original):	2
Author payment:	none
Reprints:	50 free
Time for editorial decision:	1–2 months
Time for publication of accepted manuscript:	varies
Solicited articles published per year:	50 percent
Unsolicited articles published per year:	50 percent
Acceptance rate for unsolicited articles:	not available
Refereed?	some articles are reviewed by nurse experts, but not all

Jamaican Nurse
72 Arnold Road—Mary Secole House
Kingston, 5, Jamaica, W.I.

Circulation:	4,000–5,000
Organizational association:	Nurses' Association of Jamaica
Organizational association:	3x
Yearly frequency:	2,500 words, maximum
Number of copies to submit (including original):	2
Author payment:	none
Reprints:	2 copies
Time for editorial decision:	3 months
Time for publication of accepted manuscript:	3 months
Solicited articles published per year:	15
Unsolicited articles published per year:	5
Acceptance rate for unsolicited articles:	no response

Midwife Health Visitor and Community Nurse
Recorder House
91 Stoke Newington Church Street
London, N16 OAU

Circulation:	22,000
Organizational association:	none
Yearly frequency:	12x
Average article length:	no response
Number of copies to submit (including original):	2
Author payment:	by arrangement
Reprints:	at cost
Time for editorial decision:	3 months
Time for publication of accepted manuscript:	6 months
Solicited articles published per year:	no response
Unsolicited articles published per year:	no response
Acceptance rate for unsolicited articles:	no response
Refereed?	yes

*Midwives Chronicle
98 Belsize Lane
London, NW3 5BB
England

Circulation:	19,000
Organizational association:	Royal College of Midwives
Yearly frequency:	12x
Average article length:	1,000–2,000 words
Number of copies to submit (including original):	1
Author payment:	based on length
Reprints:	at cost
Time for editorial decision:	1 week
Time for publication of accepted manuscript:	varies
Solicited articles published per year:	some
Unsolicited articles published per year:	most
Acceptance rate for unsolicited articles:	75 percent
Refereed?	yes, if the editor considers it necessary

Natnews
c/o: Newton Man Ltd.
Sherwood House
Matlock, Derbyshire, England

Circulation:	5,000
Organizational association:	National Association of Theatre Nurses
Yearly frequency:	8x
Average article length:	no regulations
Number of copies to submit (including original):	1
Author payment:	varies
Reprints:	at cost
Time for editorial decision:	2–4 weeks
Time for publication of accepted manuscript:	6–12 weeks
Solicited articles published per year:	not available
Unsolicited articles published per year:	not available
Acceptance rate for unsolicited articles:	not available

*New Zealand Nursing Journal
P.O. Box 2128
Wellington, New Zealand

Circulation:	12,739
Organizational association:	New Zealand Nurses' Assoc.
Yearly frequency:	12x
Average article length:	2,000–2,500 words
Number of copies to submit (including original):	2
Author payment:	none
Reprints:	no response
Time for editorial decision:	1 month
Time for publication of accepted manuscript:	3–6 months
Solicited articles published per year:	few
Unsolicited articles published per year:	most
Acceptance rate for unsolicited articles:	70–80 percent
Refereed?	yes

*The Nursing Journal of India
L-17, Green Park
New Delhi—110 016
India

Circulation:	14,000
Organizational association:	Trained Nurses' Association of India
Yearly frequency:	12x
Average article length:	2,000 words
Number of copies to submit (including original):	2
Author payment:	none
Reprints:	on request, at cost
Time for editorial decision:	1 month
Time for publication of accepted manuscript:	2–3 months
Solicited articles published per year:	few
Unsolicited articles published per year:	most
Acceptance rate for unsolicited articles:	50–60 percent
Refereed?	generally, manuscripts are reviewed by the editor who is also an expert in the nursing field and whenever necessary advice is also sought from the editorial board which consists of experts in various fields of nursing

Nursing Mirror
Surrey House
1, Throwley Way
Sutton, Surrey SM1 4QQ

Circulation:	57,582
Organizational association:	none
Yearly frequency:	weekly
Average article length:	2,000 words
Number of copies to submit (including original):	1
Author payment:	by negotiation
Reprints:	not supplied
Time for editorial decision:	varies
Time for publication of accepted manuscript:	varies
Solicited articles published per year:	no response
Unsolicited articles published per year:	no response
Acceptance rate for unsolicited articles:	no response
Refereed?	yes

Nursing Times
4 Little Essex Street
London, WC2 3LF
England

Circulation:	57,000
Organizational association:	none
Yearly frequency:	weekly
Average article length:	1,500–2,000 words
Number of copies to submit (including original):	2
Author payment:	by negotiation
Reprints:	at cost
Time for editorial decision:	up to 4 weeks
Time for publication of accepted manuscript:	3–6 months
Solicited articles published per year:	50 percent
Unsolicited articles published per year:	50 percent
Acceptance rate for unsolicited articles:	40 percent
Refereed?	yes

*Occupational Health
35 Red Lion Square
London, WC1R 4SG
England

Circulation:	3,700
Organizational association:	Royal College of Nursing
Yearly frequency:	12x
Average article length:	1,500–2,000 words
Number of copies to submit (including original):	2
Author payment:	by negotiation
Reprints:	6 journal copies free
Time for editorial decision:	1 month
Time for publication of accepted manuscript:	2 months
Solicited articles published per year:	50
Unsolicited articles published per year:	10
Acceptance rate for unsolicited articles:	50 percent
Refereed?	yes

World Hospitals
24 Nutford Place
London, W1H 6AN, England

Circulation:	2,500–3,500
Organizational association:	International Hospital Federation
Yearly frequency:	4x
Average article length:	3,000–5,000 words
Number of copies to submit (including original):	2
Author payment:	no response
Reprints:	at cost
Time for editorial decision:	1–3 months
Time for publication of accepted manuscript:	3–12 months
Solicited articles published per year:	6
Unsolicited articles published per year:	18
Acceptance rate for unsolicited articles:	67 percent

*Zambia Nurse
Zambia Nurses Association
Post Office Box 2104
Kitwe, Zambia

Circulation:	800
Organizational association:	Zambia Nurses Association
Yearly frequency:	3x
Average article length:	6,000–7,500 words
Number of copies to submit (including original):	no response
Author payment:	none
Reprints:	no response
Time for editorial decision:	1 month
Time for publication of accepted manuscript:	1 months
Solicited articles published per year:	varies
Unsolicited articles published per year:	most
Acceptance rate for unsolicited articles:	no response
Refereed?	varies

*The Zimbabiue-Rhodesia Nurse
Post Office Box A2
Avondale
Salisbury, Zimbabiue

Circulation:	1,000
Organizational association:	Zimbabiue Rhodesia Nurses' Association
Yearly frequency:	4x
Average article length:	250 words
Number of copies to submit (including original):	2
Author payment:	none
Reprints:	free
Time for editorial decision:	2 months
Time for publication of accepted manuscript:	3–5 months
Solicited articles published per year:	no response
Unsolicited articles published per year:	no response
Acceptance rate for unsolicited articles:	no response

LPN Journals

*The Journal of Nursing Care
265 Post Road West
Westport, CT 06880

Circulation:	70,000 plus
Organizational association:	The National Federation of Licensed Practical Nurses
Yearly frequency:	monthly
Average article length:	1,600 plus words
Number of copies to submit (including original):	no limit
Author payment:	$20.00 per page
Reprints:	none
Time for editorial decision:	one to three months
Time for publication of accepted manuscript:	two months
Solicited articles published per year:	10 articles
Unsolicited articles published per year:	65
Acceptance rate for unsolicited articles:	no response
Refereed?	yes, but editor has final say

*Journal of Practical Nursing
122 East 42nd Street (Suite 800)
New York, NY 10017

Circulation: 40,000

Organizational association: National Association for
                                      Practical Nurse Education and
                                      Service, Inc.

Yearly frequency: 12x

Average article length: 1,000–4,000 words

Number of copies to submit
(including original):   2

Author payment: usually none

Reprints: 5 journal copies free

Time for editorial decision: 6–8 weeks

Time for publication of
accepted manuscript: 2–12 months

Solicited articles
published per year: most

Unsolicited articles
published per year: some

Acceptance rate for
unsolicited articles: 35–40 percent

Refereed?   yes

Health Care Personnel

American Lung Association Bulletin
1740 Broadway
New York, NY 10019

Circulation:	40,000
Organizational association:	American Lung Association
Yearly frequency:	10x
Average article length:	2,000–2,500 words
Number of copies to submit (including original):	2
Author payment:	none
Reprints:	a reasonable number free
Time for editorial decision:	1 month maximum
Time for publication of accepted manuscript:	2–6 months
Solicited articles published per year:	60
Unsolicited articles published per year:	10
Acceptance rate for unsolicited articles:	10 percent

Critical Care Quarterly
Aspen Systems Corporation
1600 Research Blvd.
Rockville, MD 20850

Circulation:	6,066
Organizational association:	none
Yearly frequency:	quarterly
Average article length:	4,500 words
Number of copies to submit (including original):	2
Author payment:	none
Reprints:	on request for a fee
Time for editorial decision:	3–9 months
Time for publication of accepted manuscript:	3–9 months
Solicited articles published per year:	32
Unsolicited articles published per year:	8 (Note: Each issue is devoted entirely to one topic. A list of upcoming issue topics is available from the publisher.)
Refereed?	yes

*Dimensions in Health Service
Canadian Hospital Association
410 Lauvier Avenue W., Ste 800
Ottawa, K1R 7T6
Canada

Circulation:	15,000
Organizational association:	Canadian Hospital Association
Yearly frequency:	12x
Average article length:	2,000 words
Number of copies to submit (including original):	2
Author payment:	none
Reprints:	by permission only
Time for editorial decision:	minimum 1 month
Time for publication of accepted manuscript:	up to 1 year
Solicited articles published per year:	50
Unsolicited articles published per year:	50
Acceptance rate for unsolicited articles:	50 percent
Refereed?	yes

Emergency Medicine
280 Madison Avenue
New York, NY 10016

Circulation:	125,500
Organizational association:	none
Yearly frequency:	12x
Average article length:	no restriction
Number of copies to submit (including original):	1
Author payment:	none
Reprints:	100 free on request
Time for editorial decision:	1 month
Time for publication of accepted manuscript:	3 months
Solicited articles published per year:	
Unsolicited articles published per year:	most articles are staff written
Acceptance rate for unsolicited articles:	

*Family and Community Health
Aspen Systems Corporation
1600 Research Blvd.
Rockville, MD 20850

Circulation:	2,534
Organizational association:	none
Yearly frequency:	quarterly
Average article length:	4,000 words
Number of copies to submit (including original):	3
Author payment:	none
Reprints:	on request for a fee
Time for editorial decision:	8 weeks
Time for publication of accepted manuscript:	6 months
Solicited articles published per year:	35
Unsolicited articles published per year:	5 (Note: Each issue is devoted entirely to one topic. A list of upcoming issue topics is available from the publisher.)
Refereed?	yes

Family Planning Perspectives
515 Madison Avenue
New York, NY 10022

Circulation:	29,000
Organizational association:	Planned Parenthood Federation of America
Yearly frequency:	6 x
Average article length:	4,000 words
Number of copies to submit (including original):	2
Author payment:	none
Reprints:	25 free
Time for editorial decision:	1 month
Time for publication of accepted manuscript:	4 months
Solicited articles published per year:	most
Unsolicited articles published per year:	some
Acceptance rate for unsolicited articles:	10 percent

*Health Care Education
80 North Broadway
Hicksville, NY 11801

Circulation:	23,000
Organizational association:	none
Yearly frequency:	bi-monthly
Average article length:	700 words
Number of copies to submit (including original):	one
Author payment:	none
Reprints:	none
Time for editorial decision:	1–2 weeks
Time for publication of accepted manuscript:	1–3 months
Solicited articles published per year:	7
Unsolicited articles published per year:	12
Acceptance rate for unsolicited articles:	not available
Refereed?	no

Hospital and Community Psychiatry
1700 18th Street, N.W.
Washington, D.C. 20009

Circulation: 17,500

Organizational association: American Psychiatric Association

Yearly frequency: 12x

Average article length: 2,000–2,500 words

Number of copies to submit
(including original):   2

Author payment: none

Reprints: 5 journal copies free

Time for editorial decision: 2–3 months

Time for publication of
accepted manuscript: 9–12 months

Solicited articles
published per year: few

Unsolicited articles
published per year: most

Acceptance rate for
unsolicited articles: 25 percent

Hospital Formulary Management
51 E. 42nd Street
New York, NY 10017

Circulation:	25,000
Organizational association:	none
Yearly frequency:	12x
Average article length:	2,000–4,000 words
Number of copies to submit (including original):	2
Author payment:	none
Reprints:	free on request
Time for editorial decision:	1 month
Time for publication of accepted manuscript:	6 months
Solicited articles published per year:	70
Unsolicited articles published per year:	20
Acceptance rate for unsolicited articles:	50 percent

Hospital Forum
Association of Western Hospitals
830 Market Street
San Francisco, CA 94102

Circulation:	10,241
Organizational association:	Association of Western Hospitals
Yearly frequency:	12x
Average article length:	1,500–2,000 words
Number of copies to submit (including original):	2
Author payment:	none
Reprints:	depends
Time for editorial decision:	2 weeks
Time for publication of accepted manuscript:	2 months
Solicited articles published per year:	6
Unsolicited articles published per year:	30
Acceptance rate for unsolicited articles:	20 percent

Hospital Progress
1438 S. Grand Boulevard
St. Louis, MO 63104

Circulation: 16,000

Organizational association: Catholic Health Association

Yearly frequency: 12x

Average article length: 2,500–3,000 words

Number of copies to submit
(including original):   2

Author payment: by agreement

Reprints: by agreement

Time for editorial decision: 2–3 months

Time for publication of
accepted manuscript: 4 months

Solicited articles
published per year: varies

Unsolicited articles
published per year: varies

Acceptance rate for
unsolicited articles: no response

*Hospitals, Journal of the American Hospital Association
840 N. Lake Shore Drive
Chicago, IL 60611

Circulation:	75,000
Organizational association:	American Hospital Association
Yearly frequency:	24x
Average article length:	2,000–2,500 words
Number of copies to submit (including original):	3
Author payment:	usually none
Reprints:	2 journal copies free
Time for editorial decision:	2–3 months
Time for publication of accepted manuscript:	6–12 months
Solicited articles published per year:	50
Unsolicited articles published per year:	most
Acceptance rate for unsolicited articles:	20 percent
Refereed?	yes

*Journal of Allied Health
School of Allied Medical Professions
Ohio State University
1583 Perry Street
Columbus, OH 43210

Circulation:	2,500
Organizational association:	American Society of Allied Health Professions
Yearly frequency:	4x
Average article length:	up to 3,000 words
Number of copies to submit (including original):	3
Author payment:	none
Reprints:	6 journal copies free
Time for editorial decision:	2 months
Time for publication of accepted manuscript:	3–18 months
Solicited articles published per year:	0
Unsolicited articles published per year:	approximately 30
Acceptance rate for unsolicited articles:	approximately 55 percent
Refereed?	yes

*Journal of School Health
Post Office Box 708
Kent, OH 44240

Circulation:	11,000
Organizational association:	American School Health Association
Yearly frequency:	10x
Average article length:	4,000 words (maximum)
Number of copies to submit (including original):	3
Author payment:	none
Reprints:	2 journal copies free
Time for editorial decision:	2 months
Time for publication of accepted manuscript:	3–6 months
Solicited articles published per year:	0
Unsolicited articles published per year:	200
Acceptance rate for unsolicited articles:	60 percent
Refereed?	yes

Mental Hygiene
1800 N. Kent Street
Rosslyn, Arlington, VA 22209

Circulation:	7,000
Organizational association:	National Association for Mental Health
Yearly frequency:	4x
Average article length:	3,000 words
Number of copies to submit (including original):	2
Author payment:	none
Reprints:	at cost
Time for editorial decision:	3 weeks
Time for publication of accepted manuscript:	6–12 months
Solicited articles published per year:	14
Unsolicited articles published per year:	18
Acceptance rate for unsolicited articles:	12 percent

*Modern Healthcare
740 N. Rush
Chicago, IL 60611

Circulation:	52,000
Organizational association:	none
Yearly frequency:	12x
Average article length:	600–800 words
Number of copies to submit (including original):	1
Author payment:	$100
Reprints:	none
Time for editorial decision:	varies
Time for publication of accepted manuscript:	varies
Solicited articles published per year:	12
Unsolicited articles published per year:	most are staff written
Acceptance rate for unsolicited articles:	under 5 percent
Refereed?	no

P.A. *Journal*
6900 Grove Road
Thorofare, NJ 08086

Circulation:	2,800
Organizational association:	none
Yearly frequency:	4x
Average article length:	no response
Number of copies to submit (including original):	2
Author payment:	none
Reprints:	no response
Time for editorial decision:	1–2 months
Time for publication of accepted manuscript:	no response
Solicited articles published per year:	none
Unsolicited articles published per year:	30
Acceptance rate for unsolicited articles:	50 percent

Point of View
Ethicon, Inc.
Route #22
Somerville, NJ 08876

Circulation:	40,000
Organizational association:	Ethicon, Inc. (for OR, DR, ED personnel)
Yearly frequency:	4x
Average article length:	1,000–1,500 words
Number of copies to submit (including original):	2
Author payment:	$75–$150 per article
Reprints:	free
Time for editorial decision:	4–6 weeks
Time for publication of accepted manuscript:	18–24 months
Solicited articles published per year:	few
Unsolicited articles published per year:	most
Acceptance rate for unsolicited articles:	90 percent
Refereed?	yes

*Public Health Reports
10–30 Center Building
3700 East-West Highway
Hyattsville, MD 20782

Circulation:	14,000
Organizational association:	U.S. Public Health Service
Yearly frequency:	6x
Average article length:	3,000 words
Number of copies to submit (including original):	4
Author payment:	none
Reprints:	100 free to senior author
Time for editorial decision:	3–4 months
Time for publication of accepted manuscript:	6–8 months
Solicited articles published per year:	10
Unsolicited articles published per year:	80
Acceptance rate for unsolicited articles:	45 percent
Refereed?	yes

*Topics in Emergency Medicine
Aspen Systems Corporation
1600 Research Blvd.
Rockville, MD 20850

Circulation:	5,532
Organizational association:	none
Yearly frequency:	quarterly
Average article length:	4,000 words
Number of copies to submit (including original):	3
Author payment:	none
Reprints:	on request for a fee
Time for editorial decision:	8 weeks
Time for publication of accepted manuscript:	6 months
Solicited articles published per year:	35
Unsolicited articles published per year:	5 (Note: Each issue is devoted entirely to one topic. A list of upcoming issue topics is available from the publisher.)
Refereed?	yes

General Public

Family Health Magazine
1271 Avenue of the Americas
New York, NY 10020

Circulation:	1,000,000
Organizational association:	none
Yearly frequency:	12x
Average article length:	1,000–3,000 words
Number of copies to submit (including original):	1
Author payment:	depends on length and content
Reprints:	at cost
Time for editorial decision:	6 weeks
Time for publication of accepted manuscript:	varies
Solicited articles published per year:	most
Unsolicited articles published per year:	few
Acceptance rate for unsolicited articles:	very low

Life and Health
6856 Eastern Avenue, N.W.
Washington, D.C. 20012

Circulation: 100,000

Organizational association: Seventh Day Adventist Church

Yearly frequency: 12x

Average article length: 750–2,000 words

Number of copies to submit
(including original):   1

Author payment: $25–$125

Reprints: 2 journal copies free

Time for editorial decision: 2–3 months

Time for publication of
accepted manuscript: indefinite

Solicited articles
published per year: 25 percent

Unsolicited articles
published per year: 75 percent

Acceptance rate for
unsolicited articles: 10 percent

Refereed?   yes

Appendix II

Selected Readings

The following selected readings augment the content presented in the first part of the book.

"Here to There" by Art Spikol inspires appropriate use of transitions to smooth a reader's journey through your article; "Prune Your Prose" by William E. Unger, Jr., urges the elimination of verbosity; and "Are You Guilty of Murdering the English Language" by Stanley A. Chatkin encourages accurate, grammatically correct language use.

In addition, three selections provide information about the referee process for journal articles, including how it works and its significance to individual authors and the profession.

Finally, a contribution by L.E. Sissman looks at an area of writing often neglected in workshops and writing resources, but an area nurses are likely to be involved in—book reviewing. Sissman's work discusses the do's and don't's of reviewing with a focus on the moral imperatives of the task.

"HERE TO THERE"
By Art Spikol
Copyright 1979 by Art Spikol, reprinted with permission. From "Magazine Writing: The Inside Angle" (Writer's Digest Books). Published in *Writer's Digest,* 58(1):11-14, January, 1978.
Spikol is a free lance writer and regular columnist for *Writer's Digest.* His best transition occurs during lunch hour weekdays when he leaves *Philadelphia Magazine,* where he is executive editor, and walks across the street, up

one flight, to shoot pool with neophytes. He has seen "The Hustler" seventeen times.

In chapter five, "Now Write the Article," one piece of advice regarding clear writing exhorts the author to "provide transition—the bridge over all gaps." In the following article, an experienced writer/editor offers detailed information on this process—thus paving the way for a smooth reading journey, minus the "bumps" present in the work of those who leave helpless readers to find their way from thought to thought, sentence to sentence, and paragraph to paragraph.

Here to There

By Art Spikol

It's an editor's delight when an article hangs together so well that you can't find a single paragraph to eliminate. How does an article like that happen?

The secret is something called a *transition:* the passage, within a piece of writing, from one subject to another. How transitions are handled can and do make the difference in readability—because they determine how easily and naturally an article flows from paragraph to paragraph. A rough transition is like a bump; one sentence you're one place, the next sentence you're someplace else—and either you don't know what you're doing there or you're painfully *aware* of how you got there: choppy writing. Smooth transitions, on the other hand, get readers to the next subject without any awareness that the subject has changed at all; they feel that they're reading a logical extension of the previous thought. And if you've ever wondered what makes an article just plod along instead of reading quickly, chances are the article consists of paragraphs stacked one on top of another with no transitions of any kind, rough or smooth.

At their least, then, transitions get you where you want to go—and supply an apparent reason for going there. At their best, transitions make any article read like a masterpiece of logic, with one subject or avenue of thought following another so naturally, so spontaneously, it seems to the reader as if the road taken is the only plausible one to explore next.

POCKETS FULL OF MIRACLES

Perhaps the best way to show transitions in action is to go through an article, locate the transitions and see how the writer made the switch from subject to subject. To illustrate, I'll use an article about pool—pocket billiards, if you will. You aren't going to be able to read the article, but I can tell you how it came together and what happened to it along the way—how the transitions occurred.

The article opens with a good lead—enough to establish a reason for the reader to stay with it—and, shortly after the opening, takes the reader to a rather rundown pool hall. It is to be the longest scene in the story, a description which ends with this:

... And while the tables are in disrepair, the slate beds—the playing surfaces—are in decent shape. There's a lot of coming and going, but not many people hang around to shoot. Mostly, they come in to use the bathroom.

Now the transition:

You have now been to a pool hall. Let's proceed to the billiard parlors. What's the difference? The same as the difference between a housewife and a domestic engineer....

This first transition, you'll notice, is actually rather heavy handed: if you were paying attention, you felt the "bump." Fortunately, the other transitions that follow are not as obvious. Take this next one where, after talking about the generally-accepted negative image of pool halls, the paragraph *sets up* the transition that follows it:

It takes a certain amount of courage for, say, the fellow next in line for promotion to the new vice presidential slot at the insurance company to tell his gray-haired, gray-suited, gray-faced superiors that he intends to stop by the pool hall and run a few racks, and would they care to join him? But even if he has this kind of self-confidence and sense of self-worth, there is still the time-honored bugaboo: a talent at pool is the sign of a misspent youth.

Here's the next sentence—and the transition:

Actually, the game has a tradition, if not respectability, behind it. They were playing something like it in France in 1440....

At that point, the article has shifted *logically* into the origins and background of pool, and the article now traces the game from the 15th century to early 20th-century America; all of which ends with one elderly, dignified and wealthy gentleman:

... "They had high stools," he remembered, "and when I was just a young fellow, people used to come and sit on the stools and eat their lunches and watch the games."

That wraps up the history and sets us up for a description of the average pool fan—and here's the transition that gets us there:

> Most people who maintain any sort of devotion to pool usu-
> ally started out playing it in their youth, since only youth (or
> great wealth) affords the kind of free time that enables one to
> invest him/herself into the pursuit of such an unmarketable
> skill . . . .

Now follows a little more of that—the last paragraph of which naturally leads to a discussion of proficiency, like this, and again sets up a transition:

> . . . although it is certainly possible to pick up the game in
> mid-life and become proficient at it in time.

Now watch this transition immediately after the above:

> But it's not easy. The game is not simply a matter of . . .

We're smoothly into a discussion of the kind of talent it takes to shoot pool, which will take us, some paragraphs later, into a *general* discussion of those who shoot it best:

> So when you see someone shooting pool really well who looks
> really stupid, he is probably smarter than he looks, but perhaps
> took a wrong turn somewhere in life. Or a right turn, depending
> upon how you look at it.

Which leads to a *specific* discussion of those who shoot it best:

> A few of these exceptional players are known to show up at
> various Philadelphia area pool halls . . .

The article now discusses a couple of local players, including one who played against several-times world champion Luther Lassiter— a perfect opportunity to talk about the pool *halls* instead of the players, like this:

> Lassiter doesn't show up much around Philadelphia, which
> is good news for those who play the occasional tournaments at
> some of the clubs . . .

The article goes on to talk briefly about a club or two, then the piece compares the image of pool halls with the reality, winding up a description of one billiard parlor with:

> . . . and this is an extremely cordial pool hall.

Now the transition:

> Which would surprise you only if you've based your opin-
> ions on popular stereotypes, or on *The Hustler,* that 1961

movie which did for pool what *Up the Down Staircase* did for teaching . . . .

By now, the article has supplied a reason to spend quite a bit of time exploring local pool halls—and the reader has been enticed to actually want to know how these places differ from one another. Naturally, as Freud (a lousy pool shooter, incidentally) insisted, everything finally comes around to sex, and this story does, too, sliding into the subject with some talk about the more modern pool halls with their piped-in music and carpeting, and the fact that more women are frequenting pool halls these days. In fact:

If you visit the Cue and Cushion today—you will realize that nobody looks as good shooting pool as a woman.

The article talks about how women shoot pool, and how men can still beat them, and how some tired old stereotypes are still honored in certain pool-hall settings. This leads to a female psychologist claiming that the game has symbolic sexual overtones, which then leads the article into a game between two men, both of whom are interested in the same woman—a game which takes on an added import for that reason. It's a perfect way to get into pool hall gambling:

. . . Most times, of course, the stakes aren't quite so high.

Now, to complete the transition:

Ostensibly, gambling never takes place with the knowledge of the operator of the pool hall . . . .

Now the article delves into gambling—therefore, hustlers. We read about one who is quite good but not smart, and consequently doesn't make much money. The series of paragraphs ends with:

He doesn't lose, you understand, but he'll never get rich.

Which brings to the reader's mind: who *does* get rich? And not coincidentally, the next sentence is the transition:

If you could create a hustler, a bionic pool shark, he'd look like Wally Cox . . . .

The description that unfolds, of course, is a rather pointed one of a predator—and this article is, after all, a sort of upbeat one about pool. So rather than leave a wrong impression, the threat is deflated:

There are very few of these people around anymore. The ones good enough to do it lose their anonymity too quickly. So the field is glutted with amateurs . . . .

And then the article ends. We have been swept along from beginning to end.

But don't think that all of this happens simply because the writer planned it that way. An article has a life of its own, and transitions, at their best, are the natural consequences of a logical unfolding of the article. Most transitions *aren't* planned. As you write, you'll simply find yourself moving logically from one place to the next—and you won't even notice that you're writing transitions. That's what it finally comes down to: transitions are as much called for by the *story* as they are by the *author,* in the same way that once an artist starts painting, the canvas itself— the spaces still unfilled, the colors already there—tells the artist what's needed. As you read your writing, you should be able to spot only those transitions that are rough, or missing altogether. And that's when you have to build them in, create a flow that doesn't naturally exist—or, at least, didn't happen naturally.

MAKING YOUR OWN BREAKS

Let's suppose you have to go from one point to another and there just isn't any way to do it naturally. There's no logical transition staring you in the face; you're going to have to invent one. Is that OK?

Sure, as long as it doesn't *sound* invented. Remember, it shouldn't be noticeable *at all* as a writing device.

Say you've boxed yourself into a corner. You know that you've finished with the subject at hand, and now you'd like to cross the street to the next one—but damned if you can find a break in the traffic. That's where the self-contradiction (often just the word "but") comes in. You make a statement, then take exception to it. Say a paragraph ends like this:

> As the crime wave diminished, both the city and the deployment of foot patrolmen returned to normal.

That sentence has a feeling of finality about it. How are you going to (1) hold your reader, and (2) move him along to the next subject? Maybe like this:

> But—as one shopkeeper says—normal in the city is still frightening. "They say it's over," says Charlie Field, a sporting goods store owner, "but there's still a holdup a week among small businesses..."

Or:

But is normal deployment enough? Charlie Field, a sporting goods store owner, doesn't think so.

Or:

But if everything is quiet at police headquarters, it's another story at (and here you can fill in whatever you want, practically, including your own bathroom, providing the connection isn't too ridiculous).

By using these self-contradictions, the writer establishes an artificial tension that enables the article to move with impetus into the next segment. Sometimes all you have to do is *think* "but" or "despite all this" or "whether that's true or not" or a number of other variations to yield a good transitional sentence. And remember—there's nothing to stop you from going back to the previous sentence and rewriting it to *set up* a transition. Like this:

The crime wave diminished. And both the city and the police department made the mistake of thinking things were back to normal.

When you write a provocative sentence like that, you don't have to worry about a transition working; it's practically guaranteed. In fact, the next sentence could start out as innocuously as the one below and still be loaded with anticipation:

On a Saturday morning early in April, Charlie Field unlocked the door of his sporting goods store for business as usual, disarmed the burglar alarm, and threw on the lights.

Because of the setup in the previous paragraph, the reader knows something exciting is about to happen, and would actually experience a sense of disappointment if the writer didn't come through.

A thought which is, appropriately enough, a setup for another transition—mine—so excuse me while I move logically along to the Sunday *Times* crossword.

PRUNE YOUR PROSE
By William E. Unger Jr.

Copyright 1979 William E. Unger Jr. Reprinted with permission. First published by *Writer's Digest*, 59 (6): 25-26, 1979.

William E. Unger Jr. is a free-lance technical writer and editor with a Ph.D. in English. He writes for private businesses and state government committees.

> Earlier in this book, the author emphasizes the need to remove unnecessary words. The following article reinforces this cardinal rule of clarity, advising readers to apply their pruning shears to specific grammatical constructions, weak verbs, and other forms of literary weaselry.

Prune Your Prose

by William E. Unger Jr.

Are your best thoughts choking in a thicket of wordy structures? Here are some practical tips for pruning your work and making it more appealing—and salable—when you send it to an editor.

As a freelancer for business and state government agencies, I operate on the premise that, after technical competence, a writer owes the readers information presented clearly and concisely. These busy people require information they can absorb quickly and act on. The writer need not make them laugh or cry, but he must not put them to sleep.

Unfortunately, much of the prose I work with does put its readers to sleep, because it is wordy. Wordiness applies, of course, to many failings. The writer who goes on forever with nothing to say or the writer who supplies six examples where two would do nicely is being "wordy." My concern, however, is common English constructions found in sentences that must be rewritten rather than eliminated. As William Strunk wrote over 40 years ago, in his classic *Elements of Style*, "Vigorous writing is concise. A sentence should contain no unnecessary words, a paragraph no unnecessary sentences, for the same reason that a drawing should have no unnecessary lines and a machine no unnecessary parts. This requires not that a writer make all his sentences short, or that he avoid all detail and treat his subjects only in outline, but that every word tell."

Wordy structures bog down the reader and diffuse the writer's message even when unnoticed; when noticed, they cause irritation and a harsher evaluation of the product and the writer. Along with bad grammar and inappropriate dictation, wordy structures warn of trouble ahead. An editor may condescend to correct a few such structures himself, but too many of them may cause him to reject an article or return it for rewriting.

NIX SIX TICS

Various common grammatical structures almost invariably reveal wordiness. I call them "tics" because they are often written unconsciously, thus remaining uncorrected in revisions. The worst such structures are delayed subjects, prepositional phrases used as modifiers, weak verbs, the passive voice, failure to subordinate, and noun clauses containing prepositional phrases.

Perhaps the most ubiquitous writing tic is the delayed subject, the "it is" or "there are" construction so common to speech. Such a construction is almost always wordy and almost never necessary, as witness a few examples. "*It is the responsibility of the team captains* to confer with the referees" should be "The team captains are responsible for conferring with the referees." "*There are many successful novelists who* cannot write good dialogue" becomes "Many successful novelists cannot write good dialogue." "*It is obvious that there need to be representatives* from both government and industry" is much better as "Obviously, representatives from both government and industry are necessary." A writer cannot always avoid the delayed subject, but he should cultivate the habit of peering at it suspiciously whenever he writes it.

For reasons that mystify me, many writers avoid using possessives and other immediate modifiers. Instead, they employ prepositional phrases and relative clauses, thereby losing clarity and conciseness. I frequently read such constructions as "*the goals and objectives of the writer*" or "*since the inception of the magazine*" instead of "the writer's goals and objectives" or "the magazine's inception." Sentences such as "Studies indicate that *workers who are self motivated* produce more" are common, whereas "self-motivated workers" does better in every respect.

WEAK VERBS AND WEASELRY

Weak verbs are the lazy writer's crutch and the reader's despair. Forms of the verbs *to be* and *to have* should function primarily as helping verbs. They lack the vigor to carry the full weight of most sentences; often when a writer tries to make them do so, he must supply a noun clause to complete his thought. Usually a verb equivalent for the noun in the clause can replace the whole string of words. Sometimes the verb *to make* also functions like the verb *to be*.

I find constructions like the following everywhere: "the move toward eliminating freelance materials *was a result of a change* in the editor's policy"; "to meet the deadline, we must *have the completed drafts done* early"; "he will be able *to make an intelligent decision about what jobs* to undertake"; "because the change *will be profitable for everyone*." The careful writer will examine his work for weak verbs and prune all he can: "the move toward eliminating free-lance material resulted from a change in the editor's policy"; "to meet the deadline, we must complete the drafts early"; "he will be able to decide intelligently. . ."; "because the change will profit everyone."

The basic English sentence is active; it moves from actor, through action (the verb), to object. The passive reverses this order, placing the object first, diffusing the action by combining the verb's past participle with a form of *to be*, and ending with the actor, or omitting the actor completely. The passive voice has two serious defects. It lends itself to "weaselry," or avoiding responsibility ("*It is widely held that*" translates as "I believe"), and it provides a splendid opportunity to use more words with less clarity. The active voice gives life to the English language, but many writers shy away from it, probably feeling that "I" will somehow seem egotistical (even if they have obviously done the work and their opinions will be evaluated). I think such a philosophy is nonsense; however, I recognize that some companies, for instance, may require the authors of public documents to remain in the background, preferring to imply the company as author rather than any individual.

The following sentences appeared in a business analysis: "The discussion here *will be focused* on these changes and an explanation as to why they have occurred, employing the resource-dependency conceptual framework of organization-environmental relationships. Also *included will be* an examination of the degrees to which different organizations are implementing these changes and an explanation as to why these variances exist." To keep the reader awake, pruning is clearly required; even if the jargon must remain, responsibility and conciseness both demand the active voice: "I will discuss these changes and explain why they have occurred, employing. . . . I will also examine the degree to which . . . and explain why these variances exist."

PRUNING THE PRODUCT

Often, however, a writer can eliminate the passive, and thus wordiness, without using the first person. "*It can be seen that* in the problem now *faced by* the company, the standards of desired behavior are ambiguous" should simply read, "In the problem the company now faces." "By raising Jones to a management level, the required interaction between the two departments *can be more readily assured*" is easily rewritten as "Raising Jones to a management level will more readily assure the required interaction . . ."

Failure to subordinate can lead to wordiness and dull prose. If most of a writer's sentences are short, simple statements and especially if he finds himself starting a sentence with the same noun that ended the previous sentence or with a pronoun referring to it, he should consider subordination to eliminate wordiness and to vary his style. I often encounter sentences like the following: "The science fiction novel permits a writer to answer a 'what if' question. *In this novel, the question is what if the South had won the Civil War.*" Much is gained by rewriting to "The science fiction novel permits . . . question—what if the South had won the Civil War in this particular novel." Another common construction: "This detective story takes place in three main locations. *They are Istanbul, New York and Paris.*" Here the colon is useful. "This detective story . . . locations: Istanbul, New York and Paris." ("This detective story takes place in Istanbul, New York and Paris" is even better.)

Finally, every writer should carefully reread his copy looking for subjects and objects that consist of noun clauses containing prepositional phrases. They are usually wordy and awkward, as in "*The completion of* this novel will lead to significant opportunities for Ms. Smith" or "*The use of* an electric typewriter and *the purchase of* paper in bulk can save time and money." Gerunds should replace these common constructions: "completing this novel" and "using an electric typewriter and buying paper in bulk."

I have spent considerable time, for which I was well paid, chopping at manuscripts whose every sentence seemed to contain one or more of the problems I've discussed here. (If I *hadn't* been well paid, I would have quickly written "unacceptable" on them and gone on to something more entertaining.) In fact, I pruned several wordy constructions from my first draft. Every writer must remain aware of them and must rewrite—sometimes easier said than done.

A sentence from a recent *WD* article on English usage illustrates how even a professional writer concerned with language may occasionally slip in this regard: "It is a rule of English that the plural is formed by the addition of 's'." In one short sentence, the author managed to construct a delayed subject, a passive voice, and an "of...the" noun clause. Since the sentence is totally prescriptive in any case, I submit that nothing is lost and much is gained—in addition to eliminating nine words—by rewriting it to read: "English forms the plural by adding 's'."

I have pruned a total of 63 words in my sample revisions, at least a paragraph's worth of obstruction, and 23 percent deadwood. Whether the writer is correcting his own work to make it more salable or is turning someone else's work into an acceptable product, the ability to recognize and eliminate wordy structures is a skill well worth possessing.

"ARE YOU GUILTY OF MURDERING THE ENGLISH LANGUAGE?"

by Stanley A. Chatkin

Stanley A. Chatkin, from Forest Hills, New York, has written/produced industrial films, written for *Cracked* magazine and numerous trade magazines, and has said "you know" only four times in his life.

Painlessly heighten your awareness of common grammatical errors and language misuse by reading this entertaining article and taking the incorporated test.

Go ahead—chuckle through Chatkin's exercise and emerge with raised consciousness and increased ability to use words accurately and apply established rules of grammar.

Are You Guilty of Murdering the English Language?

by Stanley A. Chatkin

Many of us learned English composition way back in the dark ages when accurate expression of thought was still a sacrosanct objective. We were trained to observe strict rules of grammar and to employ words in their true sense. But today, sadly, verbal communication has deteriorated from precise to clumsy, from definitive to vague, from proper to sloppy.

To dramatize the point, let us eavesdrop on two young secretaries riding the bus to work one morning:

"How do you like your new job?"

"Well, my boss, you know, freaks me out. Right? He's very nice, though. A very together person. I really know where his head is at."

"Does he let you do your own thing?"

"Yeah. Every one of us can work their own way. He's very easy on the other girls and myself. And as head of the company, I expected him, you know, to be a lot stricter."

"I wish my boss was like that. Like, um, he's always uptight on account of my coming in late. He's very into fund raising and gives me a large amount of letters to type. But the view from the office, oh wow. You can see the whole skyline looking out the window. Up so high, you can feel nauseous."

"My desk is in the hall; I don't have no window. But it's a swell job, irregardless. Well, here's where I get off. I'll contact ya later. Stay cool."

Any dynamic language will justifiably evolve to meet the changing needs of its society. But we must never allow properly-established definitions of words and rules of grammar to be watered down or corrupted for any reason, especially apathy or laziness. Yet English is being slowly murdered.

Nearly everywhere these days—in literature, on radio and television, in the speech of ordinary persons and famous orators alike—we are bombarded with garbled grammar and doltish diction. The principles of good English are all but ignored, and careful wording falls under the heels of puerile crudities and invalid neologisms. *We are even told, by those who should know better, that inarticulate communication is entirely permissible, just so long as the other person knows what we are talking about!*

Are you an accomplice to the crime? Let's see. The following paragraphs contain forty examples of frequent errors in grammar, syntax and diction. Can you find them? Take ye and read with blue pencil in hand:

Just between you and I, everyone should finalize their education; and hopefully you agree. If you will contact Tom or myself, we'll loan you the tuition to return to school and improve your competency. You should do this, even if you only take one course at a time like Tom and me did.

More importantly, such action is viable and healthy for you, especially in this technological age. Even the news media says so. With a good education under your belt, you will be fulfilled. People will know where you're coming from, and you'll be able to do your own thing. But don't feel badly if you haven't finished school, for you can always do that. Just remember that a man who is educated is different than one who is not. And also, knowledge is relevant and helps you to cope.

For example, I have a friend that lives down the street named Harold. He enjoys less outside activities than others do; but irregardless of his quiet life, he is a together person.

Sinking in the west one evening, Harold watched the sun disappear below the horizon; and he murmured, "I wonder where it's at now?" So he snuck a look at a textbook and then joined a class of fifty students. Today he is one of the most unique astronomers in the world.

Anyone with smarts should opt for as much education as possible. The reason is because your life will be more meaningful as your knowledge increases. As President of the United States, I think Jimmy Carter should encourage all of us to go on learning.

For corrections and explanations, read on.

ANSWERS TO TEST:

Just between you and me, everyone should complete his education; and it is hoped that you agree. If you will call Tom or me, we'll lend you the tuition to return to school and improve your competence. You should do this, even if you take only one course at a time as Tom and I did.

More important such action is beneficial and healthful for you, especially in this technologic age. Even the news media say so. With a good education under your belt, you will find satisfaction. People will respect your authority, and you will be able to live your life as you wish. But don't feel bad if you haven't finished school, for you can always do that. Just remember that a man who is educated is different from one who is not. Also, knowledge is relevant to success and helps you to cope with life's problems.

For example, I have a friend named Harold, who lives down the street. He enjoys fewer outside activities than others do; but regardless of his quiet life, he is a substantial person.

One evening, Harold watched the sun sink in the west, then disappear below the horizon; and he murmured, "I wonder where it is now." So he sneaked a look at a textbook and then joined a class of fifty pupils. Today he is one of the most respected astronomers in the world.

Anyone with intelligence should strive for as much education as possible. The reason is that your life will be more productive as your knowledge increases. I think that Jimmy Carter, as President of the United States, should encourage all of us to go on learning.

EXPLANATIONS:

1. *Me* is the object of a preposition.
2. *Finalize* is not (and has no right to be) an accepted neologism. *Complete* is more descriptive.
3. NEVER use a plural pronoun to agree with a singular antecedent. In this context, *his* is totally asexual and has always been correct, despite the insistence of women's libbers.
4. Will the agreement, itself, be hopeful? Of course not. The writer hopes for an agreement.
5. You contact someone by physically touching him. In the context of this sentence, it is preferable to call him or write to him.
6. *Myself* denotes a reflexive action, which this is not. *Me* is the object of an action by someone else.

7. *Loan* is a noun: I want a loan. How much will you lend me?
8. Why create a noun from an already-existing noun? From the adjective, *competent,* we derive the noun, *competence.* There is no need to complicate matters by adding a *y.*
9. Ah, the ubiquitous misplaced *only!* If he *only takes* one course, he will do nothing else: He will not eat, sleep, talk, etc. But if he *takes only* one course, we know without question he is limiting his study to one subject.
10. Please do not be misled by Madison Avenue illiterates. *As* is used when it is followed by a noun or pronoun and a verb. *Like* is used when it is followed only by a noun or pronoun.
11. *I* is the nominative case, not the objective.
12. An adjective, not an adverb, is needed here. Besides, there is no such word as *importantly.*
13. The proper definition of *viable* is "capable of growth." Children are viable. So are tulip bulbs. But action is not.
14. You are *healthy* (in a state of health). The action is *healthful* (promoting health).
15. Why create an adjective from an already-existing adjective? From the noun, *technology,* we derive the adjective, *technologic.* The -*al* suffix is redundant.
16. *Media* is a plural noun and requires a plural verb.
17. A hope, or a dream, or a goal is *fulfilled.* A person is not.
18. We know "where you're coming from" only if you tell us that you are, at this very moment, enroute from Chicago to New Orleans. Otherwise, the phrase, as used in its current vernacular, is crudity at its worst.
19. "Do your own thing" lacks clarity. It tells little, if anything.
20. One feels *badly* with his hands. Emotionally, he feels *bad.*
21. *Different than* denotes literary incompetence and is never correct except in this construction: George is different from Harvey, but Fred is even more *different than* George (is from Harvey).
22. *And also* is redundant. Choose one word or the other.
23. Relevant to *what?* This word cannot stand alone. There must be a comparison of some kind.
24. Cope with *what?* Like *relevant, cope* cannot stand alone. This verb is not totally intransitive. One must cope *with* something.
25. Is the street named Harold, or is the friend? Beware the dan-

gling modifier.

26.   *Who* applies to a person. *That* denotes an inanimate object.

27.   *Less* is qualitative; *fewer* is quantitative: There is *less* education in the schools today because of *fewer* dedicated teachers.

28.   *Irregardless,* obviously, is a double negative.

29.   *Together,* in this context, is ludicrous and tells nothing except that the writer is a dolt. A person cannot be described as *together,* unless it must be indicated that he has not been dismembered.

30.   Did Harold sink in the west, or did the sun? Dangling participle.

31.   *At* is unnecessary and is in poor taste.

32.   A sentence beginning, "I wonder..." is declarative and does not require a question mark. An exception is, "I wonder: where is it?"

33.   There is no such word as *snuck*.

34.   Were all of them students? Hardly. All were pupils. Only some were students. Every enrollee is a pupil; but only one who studies is a student.

35.   There are no degrees of uniqueness. Either one is unique, or he is not.

36.   *Smart* is an adjective, not a noun. To use it as a noun is a sign of carelessness. (But *smart* can be used an an intransitive verb, meaning "to sting.")

37.   *Opt* is a stupid Madison Avenue contrivance. Why bother with it?

38.   *Reason is because* is never correct. We may say either, "Suzie failed the exam *because* she did not study," or "The reason Suzie failed is *that* she did not study."

39.   *Meaningful* is a lazy man's word that lacks clear connotation. Be more precise.

40.   Who is the President? The writer or Jimmy Carter? Dangling modifier.

RATE YOURSELF:

Count the errors you detected and multiply the total by 2.5. A perfect score is 100.

100 Sign your name Webster Roget, Esq.

90-99 Professor Emeritus at Oxford University
80-89 Serious, careful grammarian
70-79 Somewhat negligent in clarity and construction
60-69 Average, sloppy, careless writer
50-59 High school dropout
40-49 Radio or television commentator
30-39 Advertising copywriter
 0-29 Return to kindergarten. And this time, pay attention!

THE "REFEREE" ISSUE

Within nursing, the debate over the significance of publishing in "refereed" journals and the importance of the refereed journal to the profession's development, is becoming increasingly lively. Nurse authors need to consider all sides of this issue and determine whether it is never, sometimes, usually, or always important for them to publish in refereed journals.

What makes a "refereed" journal different from a "non-refereed" one? Definitions vary, but basically, when a journal is refereed, experts in a particular field who are not part of the editorial staff review articles and contribute to decisions regarding acceptance, rejection, or recommendations for revision. To help readers better understand the referee issue, three selections are reprinted here. "Working With Referees", a chapter from the book *The Scientist As Editor* by M. O'Connor, provides detailed information on how refereeing works. The reprinted editorial, "A Peerless Publication" by Edith P. Lewis, former editor of *Nursing Outlook,* and a response to that editorial by Helen K. Grace, dean, College of Nursing, University of Illinois, highlight the advantages and disadvantages of the referee process. The authors focus on the role of the refereed journal in the development of a discipline's body of knowledge as well as the importance of publishing in refereed journals to individuals.

"WORKING WITH REFEREES"

Chapter from O'Connor, M. *The Scientist as Editor.* New York: John Wiley and Sons, Inc., 1979, pp. 28-40. Reprinted with permission of Pitman Medical Limited, Tunbridge Wells, Kent, England (first publisher) and the author.
Maeve O'Connor is Senior Editor, Ciba Foundation, London.

Working with Referees
by M. O'Connor

Refereeing of unsolicited articles submitted to journals is the main topic of this selection. Refereeing of solicited papers for books or journals is dealt with briefly. Alternatives to refereeing are also discussed.

WHAT DO REFEREES DO?

The main function of referees is to advise editors—*not* decide for them—whether papers are suitable for publication *in a particular journal,* and whether the work is original, of high quality, up to date, and described in sufficient detail and clearly enough for readers to follow the argument or replicate the procedures discussed. This system of peer review is usually regarded as the lynchpin of reliable scientific publication, yet there is no rigorous proof of its efficacy[1] and it is attacked for the anonymity that referees often enjoy, for delaying publication, and for being elitist, conservative and conducive to plagiarism. The system is an acknowledgment that not all editors can be polymaths: most need advice about work on the periphery of their specialties, and many have to be rescued either from accepting articles that are brilliant but unsuitable for their journals or from rejecting those that are important but badly written.

Refereeing is commonly thought to be simply a matter of accepting or rejecting papers, but it is more than that. Referees also help editors to educate authors by suggesting improvements in the form and presentation of papers. Most authors respond well to constructive criticism or advice, especially as they usually have to act on it before they can get their work published. The comments they receive from editors and referees may help them when they write their next papers, and in the long run the load on editors and referees should be gradually lightened.

In some countries and disciplines the refereeing system is not as highly developed as in others. Editors who decide to adopt stricter criteria must not suddenly start rejecting every paper that fails to match the new standards. A single unconventional paper may be worth several based on competent and well-presented research. Editors and referees must learn to distinguish between unorthodox but brilliant papers and those containing statements or conclusions that are wrong, trivial or based on inadequate methods.

HOW MANY REFEREES, WHO ARE THEY, AND HOW DO THEY WORK?

Whether editors use one, two, or more referees for each paper is a matter of choice, not an unvarying rule. Two is the commonest number. The more there are, the longer the process is likely to take, unless editors stick to very firm schedules.

Referees may be members of the editorial board, associate editors, or others representing the disciplines covered by the journal. Ideally they should know their subject in depth but not be narrowly confined to one topic; be fair to authors and readers alike; have high standards but be generous towards minor flaws; be conscientious but not nitpicking; be prompt in returning manuscripts but not superficial in assessing them; and possess impeccably sound judgment. Such paragons are rare, but with the two-referee system editors can compare one referee's report with another's and gradually identify referees who have many of the good qualities and few of the bad[2]. If this comparison shows that some referees make assessments that are often wrong or prejudiced, the editor should remove them from the journal's list of advisers. Referees who constantly recommend papers that are later justly criticized by readers should be dropped too[3], since soundness of judgment cannot be taught. Slowness is another incurable habit and referees who hold manuscripts longer than the scheduled time more than twice in succession should also be struck off the list. Prejudice can be compensated for, and fairness encouraged, by the guidance the editor gives to referees.

The choice of referees does not always fall entirely on the editor's shoulders. Some editors invite authors to take part in the selection. For example, the *Proceedings of the National Academy of Sciences, USA* has a system of 'pre-review' by which authors can submit manuscripts through any member of the Academy who is willing to consider them. If the paper appears likely to deserve publication, the Academy then selects two referees who are experts in the field. If the referees approve of the manuscript, it is forwarded with their comments and those of the Academy member to the Editorial Office, with a recommendation that the manuscript be published. Even if one referee advises against acceptance, the Academy member has the right to recommend that this advice be overruled, and to explain why, if the member and the other referee favour publication. In such cases publication usually follows more or less automatically, although the Managing Editor, and the Chairman of the Editorial Board reserve the right to ask the Academy member to reconsider such a recommendation. Sometimes they may even reject the paper, but this rarely happens. The Academy member's name appears on the published article as 'Communicator' and members therefore take this responsibility very seriously—though they themselves can have papers published in the *Proceedings* without any refereeing, if they wish. The system is particularly suitable for a journal of wide scope, since the editor in effect delegates the choice of referees to someone working in the same field as the author.

In another system, used by the *Journal of Biological Chemistry* and others, all papers submitted go first to the editorial office, where each is assigned to an Associate Editor or to the Editor-in-Chief. The Editor or Associate Editor then assigns the paper to a member of the Editorial Board who is considered especially competent to deal with it, or the Associate Editor may handle the paper directly. The Editorial Board member (or the Associate Editor) may consult referees, if necessary, but does not have to do so. The Board member's decision letter, often with referees' reports or extracts from them, goes to the Associate Editor, who may revise the letter slightly before sending it to the author, usually with any referees' reports. If the Board member has recommended rejection, the manuscript goes to another Board member, or occasionally to more than one, and the procedure just described is repeated. If revision is requested, the author returns the revised manuscript directly to the Associate Editor, not to the editorial office. The Associate Editor has full authority to accept the paper; if this happens, the manuscript goes back to the editorial office, its arrival is recorded and it is sent on to the copy editors before being passed for printing. In this system, authors do not choose the Associate Editors who will handle their papers, though they may express a preference when they submit their papers. Although the system introduces an extra step in handling, it allows the editorial office to spread the work evenly between the available Associate Editors.

Another variant is for a small core of local Associate Editors (say five to seven) to meet weekly or fortnightly to discuss each manuscript and the comments made on it by outside referees as well as by one of the Associate Editors. This system seems cumbersome and liable to lead to superficial judgments taken under pressure of time and personality but where it is used it is apparently much enjoyed by the committee members for its educational value, and it often leads more naturally than other systems to the emergence of a successor to the chief editor when a term of office ends.

WHY DO REFEREES REFEREE?

Refereeing is time-consuming and often troublesome, it provides its practitioners with little public recognition and even less money, and it leaves them open to the charges of conservatism and plagiarism. Yet it is surprisingly easy, especially for an established journal, for editors to enlist referees of high standing. Many scientists look on the work as part of their wider obligation to science. Many even regard their selection as an honour, or at least as potentially useful to their careers. Others agree to be referees for the educational benefits it brings them: they see the most up-to-date information in their subject well before it is published, and they also learn something from reading the editor's comments and those of any other referees who review the same manuscript.

Many people therefore accept an invitation to join a panel of referees with little hesitation. Keeping them happy on that panel is another matter. If the editor understands people's motives for being referees, several things can be done to reward them for their work.

One is to publish, at the end of each year, a list of referees who have acted for the journal during the year. Another is to let it be known that appointments to the editorial board—which provide visible evidence of scientific status—are made from the ranks of referees whose work has been particularly valuable. A third way is to keep referees informed about what happens to the manuscripts they work on, sending them copies of other referees' comments and of letters of decision to authors; and if the editor has acted against a referee's advice, a letter of explanation is usually appreciated. These communications take a little time, and increase the costs of photocopying and postage, but the rewards in goodwill are great.

Monetary rewards for referees are rare. Where payment is made it is usually intended to cover not much more than postage costs. Few scientific journals could survive financially if they had to pay their referees at a rate commensurate with the time spent. And, in spite of what some people think, 'commercial' journals are in no better position to pay for such work than are journals sponsored by societies or institutions.

GUIDELINES FOR REFEREES

Since different journals have different specific requirements, it is as well for each to have printed guidelines, stating the journal's policy and telling referees what kind of papers to look for and what kind of information the editor wants[4]. Referees should be told:

(1) That they are allowed to refuse to review a manuscript without giving reasons;
(2) That they are the editor's advisers, not the final arbiters;
(3) Whether they should comment on presentation or only on content (to the extent that these can be separated).

They should also be asked:

(4) Do the data support the conclusions?
(5) Do any parts of the paper call for elaboration, clarification or condensation?
(6) Are the title and abstract fully informative and do they accurately reflect the content of the paper?

(7) Are there errors in computation, equations, formulae, derivations, tables, graphs or drawings, or nomenclature?

(8) Is the number of references excessive?

Many journals also provide a standard form, incorporating some of these questions, for referees' reports. Since not everyone likes these forms, referees should be told whether it is essential to fill them in or whether other ways of commenting are sufficient.

Lastly, referees should be asked not to correspond directly with the authors, and the journal's policy on anonymity of review should be stated.

REFEREEING PROCEDURES

There are almost as many variations in refereeing systems as there are journals using them. Whatever system the journal adopts, flexibility is recommended: for example, if it is obvious that a particular manuscript needs no refereeing, the editor should simply accept it for publication, or reject it, as the case may be. If this attitude conflicts with the policies of the journal's sponsor, the editor has to try to convince the sponsor of the advantages of flexibility.

Depending on which variant of the refereeing system a journal prefers, the editor deals with manuscripts after their arrival has been recorded and acknowledged basically as follows.

(1) Manuscripts are assigned to one of three categories: accepted, rejected, and for refereeing—the last being the largest category.

(2) Accepted manuscripts are kept for editing and copy-editing, and acceptance letters are sent to the authors. Rejected manuscripts are returned to the authors, with tactful letters explaining why they are not suitable for publication in the journal and possibly suggesting other journals to which the papers might be submitted.

(3) One or more referees are selected for each manuscript that is to be refereed. A copy of the manuscript is sent to each referee selected, together with the guidelines for referees and the form for comments.

(4) If a paper is to go to two referees one of the following four procedures, or something similar, can be used:

    (a) A copy can be sent to both referees simultaneously, perhaps after a telephone call to make sure that they are willing and available. When comments arrive they are compared and any contradictions are dealt with.

or (b) A member of the editorial board may be sent two copies of the manuscript and asked to select a second referee or to select two referees. The board member can be asked either to collate the two reviews and draft a letter to the author for the editor's consideration, or to send reviews straight to the editor.

or (c) The manuscript can be sent to one referee and, when the review is returned, the manuscript can be sent to a second referee selected either because the editor wants advice on an aspect not dealt with adequately by the first referee, or because the editor wants to counterbalance what looks like bias in the first review. A copy of the first review may or may not be sent to the second referee with the manuscript, as seems appropriate.

or (d) If only one referee is generally consulted, a variant of 4(a), (b), or (c) may nevertheless be used when a manuscript has too many facets for one referee to cope with.

(5) A referee's review (and the manuscript, if its return is requested) should be acknowledged as soon as it reaches the editorial office. If no review arrives by the date requested, a telephone call or a reminder card is sent to the referee. If the review still doesn't arrive, the editor telephones or cables for an answer, or proceeds without the review, according to the established policy of the journal.

(6) When the editor has read the review(s) and decided whether to accept a manuscript outright, to accept or reconsider it subject to revision, or to reject it, an appropriate letter is sent to the author. Constructive suggestions for changes or concrete reasons for rejection are given in the letter. Any abrasive comments by referees are toned down without the basic criticism being removed (and the editor may want to tell the referee why this has been done, as mentioned earlier). Except as noted in

(7) below, the referees are sent copies of the editor's letters to authors.

(7)   If the author is asked to revise the paper, the editor writes to the referees after the revised manuscript has arrived and a further decision has been made about it. The editor may be able to accept the revised version without sending it to the referee(s) again; but if major revision was requested and the editor cannot judge whether the referees' criticisms have been met, or if the author provides detailed rebuttals of the criticisms, the revised manuscript and the author's comments are sent to one or both of the original referees. When a final decision has been reached, the editor thanks the referees and sends them copies of the relevant letters and comments.

(8)   If the author has not replied to a request for revision after about six months, the correspondence is reviewed. It may be worth writing a follow-up letter, as a show of interest in the paper may bring it in even after such a long delay. If no reply appears after another six to eight weeks it is probably safe to assume that the author is not going to produce a revised manuscript. The editor then marks the folder PRESUME WITH-DRAWN and moves it out of the PENDING file.

RECONCILING CONFLICTING OPINIONS

If two referees of similar expertise and status disagree about the acceptability of a manuscript or the need for revision, the editor has to find some way of reconciling their verdicts. If the 'negative' referee is criticizing what the paper does *not* do—the approaches to the problem which the author might have used but didn't, the extra experiments which might be valuable but are not needed to validate the conclusions—the editor may choose to disregard the advice, since the referee should simply have judged the paper as submitted. On the other hand, if the 'positive' referee seems to have been superficial and to have overlooked the deficiencies pointed out by the other referee, the editor may disregard the 'positive' decision. If the editor's knowledge of the subject is sketchy, the 'positive' referee may be sent a copy of the 'negative' report (with or without being told who wrote it) and asked to say frankly whether it seems valid.

If there are differences of opinion about revision, the editor is probably the best judge of which suggestions for revision are reasonable. The suggestions should be made as specific as possible and the author should be told which revisions are considered essential, which are not essential but important, and which are optional for acceptability.

Another way of reaching a decision when referees disagree is to send the paper to one or two new referees, after telling them about the reactions already received. The value of increasing the number of advisers is, however, somewhat doubtful. As Ingelfinger[5] points out, referees' opinions are highly variable and there is no reason why the opinion of referee 3 should carry any more weight than that of referee 1 or 2. Rather than obtaining a third review, a better course is to ask a final adviser not to arbitrate but to comment on the reviews as well as on the manuscript. This really should give the editor the information needed to reach a sensible decision.

A fourth method is to follow the dictum: 'If referees differ violently, publish the paper; there must be something exciting in it.'

THE CHARGES AGAINST REFEREEING

In any discussion of refereeing, anonymity is the first aspect attacked. The other main charges are that referees tend to be conservative and elitist, that they delay publication unnecessarily, and that they can plagiarize all too easily.

Anonymity

Most editors decide after careful consideration of the pros and cons that referees' identities should not be made known to the author[6]. But if a referee firmly believes that reports should be signed, this should be allowed, even if the general policy of the journal is to keep its referees anonymous. Similarly, a referee who insists on remaining anonymous should be allowed to do so even if the journal usually sends signed reports to authors.

The question of anonymity surfaces regularly in the correspondence columns of journals and it is often suggested that, if referees are to remain anonymous, the names of authors should in all fairness be concealed from the referees. The argument is that when referees

see the title page they may be biased either in favour of the manuscript or against it, depending on whether the paper comes from a
prestigious author or department or from an unknown author at an
obscure institution, or (perhaps worst) from a rival in the field. But
removing the title page does little to hide the laboratory of origin
from knowledgeable referees, or referees may spend more time
guessing who the authors are than considering the content of the
manuscript.

Ill-feeling is inevitable if referees are outspoken in their criticism
of poor work, and referees must be protected from authors' reactions. The editor must, however, also be careful to protect the authors by detecting and suppressing biased and unjustified criticism
when it occurs. This does not mean that the criticism should be sup-
pressed when the paper is rejected: editors who reject papers without
giving reasons are behaving as though they were infallible; conversely, if they think their reasons will not withstand scrutiny, they
have no basis for rejecting those papers. Openness with authors,
while hardly the royal road to popularity, is the best policy in the end,
even though the cloak of 'confidentiality' under which some editors
shelter may seem to protect them from trouble in the short term.

A related question is whether referees of the same papers should be
identified to each other. Here, identification probably does more
good than harm. It is likely to make referees less prone to carelessness
and capriciousness.

Conservatism and elitism

Referees are chosen for their expert knowledge. This very expertise
tends to make them partial to a particular way of looking at a
subject—although top-flight scientists are (by definition) open to
new views and ready to see dogma shattered. Most referees are probably in the very good but not top category, largely because the most
senior scientists are too busy to review papers promptly. Editors
should therefore watch for excessive conservatism and try to coun-
teract it by accepting unorthodox papers if they seem methodologi-
cally sound, even if the referees have advised that the conclusions
differ from the current consensus. Instinct, and the general criteria
of scientific method, help editors to distinguish unorthodox, sound

papers from unorthodox, unsound papers. Outside advice is surely not needed to tell an editor whether the observations are too few to support the conclusions, the statistical methods weak or inappropriate, or the data internally inconsistent. The editor may indeed be more objective than a specialist referee when the results obtained are contrary to cherished current beliefs.

Commentators in various disciplines—for example, Neufeld in physics[7]; DeBakey and Pyke in biomedicine[8,9]—have pointed out that referees tend to be biased in favour of rejection, and they suggest that the editor should compensate for this. Appropriately worded guidelines are one way of counteracting this bias.

Delays and plagiarism

Referees are sometimes accused of delaying publication while they incorporate the results or methods of the refereed work into their own research or publications. This of course is conscious plagiarism; it is rare because it is easily exposed and always condemned, however distinguished the plagiarist. Authors who are worried about plagiarism by referees can protect themselves by presenting their work at seminars and conferences before submitting a paper for publication. At these meetings they not only announce their work but may also receive valuable criticism. Another suggestion[10] is that abstracts of submitted articles should be published in an abstracts journal as evidence of authorship of an idea or conclusion. Such a system would, however, be open to abuse by authors, who could stake out intellectual ground to which they had little or no title. In addition, a high proportion of 'abstracts' published before conferences—and perhaps better called 'synopses' in these circumstances—are never substantiated in published articles, either because the authors describe studies that do not survive further work and critical scrutiny, or simply because the authors never find time to finish the work as planned.

Editors can circumvent the problem of plagiarism, as well as the general charge of delay, by insisting on rapid refereeing, say within two to three weeks (though a determined plagiarist could still delay publication by providing a review full of minor criticisms and suggestions for revision). Referees can be asked to return manuscripts *im-*

mediately if they know they cannot meet the deadline or if a particular manuscript is too close to their own current work, or for any other reason, including fear of unconscious plagiarism. Better still, if the journal's budget permits, is for the editor to telephone referees first to make sure that they will accept the manuscript and can do the work within the time specified. Another device is to attach a sticker to the envelope, asking the addressee's secretary to return the packet if the referee is out of town; a covering note to the same effect can be enclosed in case the sticker is overlooked.

Delay can also be reduced by careful choice of referees. On a file card for each referee the time spent on each previously reviewed manuscript should be recorded. The card also shows whether that referee has recently been sent any manuscripts for review, though it will not show how much other work, including manuscripts from other journals, the referee has on hand. A fairer method may be to send manuscripts only to members of the editorial board, with members being invited to join the board on the strict understanding that they will receive no more than an agreed number of manuscripts for refereeing in any one year. Clear, succinct guidelines for the referee to work from also help to reduce delay. Lastly, referees' time should not be wasted with papers the editor can handle without their advice.

Of course, when authors revise papers they often introduce much longer delays than referees ever do. Some of the criticisms about delay being caused by referees can be forestalled if the date of receipt, including receipt of a revised version, and the date of acceptance are printed in the published papers. Publication of these dates has more implications for claims to priority than may be realized at first[11].

ALTERNATIVES TO REFEREEING

The alternatives to a full refereeing system are (a) no refereeing at all—which means selection by the editor alone, with or without improvement of the presentation; (b) refereeing of certain topics only; (c) refereeing of borderline manuscripts only; and (d) refereeing of only those manuscripts that—though clearly acceptable—need expert polishing.

(a) The advantage of using no referees is speed of decision; the disadvantage, the risk of a wrong decision. If an editor's most frequent mistake is to reject good papers, science is not necessarily any worse off: the authors will simply submit their papers to other journals and probably get them published. The first journal may miss some good papers but there may be enough good ones around for this not to matter much.

If an editor's most frequent mistake is to publish papers that are not up to standard, the journal's correspondents will soon comment on this. The editor either learns from those mistakes or decides to consult referees in the future.

When no referees are consulted editors are perhaps justified in giving no reason, apart from lack of space, for refusing papers; they are probably not in a strong position to provide expert criticism except in limited areas of their subjects, and to offer an elementary critique of scientific method may be insulting after what has obviously been a hurried reading. Authors who submit manuscripts to journals that do not use referees probably expect summary acceptance or rejection. If papers are accepted, authors are entitled to expect some editorial help with presentation, e.g. clarification or condensation, improvement of terminology or help with illustrations, if such help is not provided, they may well prefer to send their manuscripts to a 'Letters' journal whose sole purpose is rapid publication.

(b) Refereeing of certain topics only is a useful way of dealing with aspects of the field which lie outside the editor's experience or competence.

(c) Refereeing of borderline papers only is a good way of applying the educational function of the refereeing system where it is most needed. This procedure will cater for manuscripts from inexperienced or scientifically isolated authors who hope to get advice from more experienced workers than those with whom they are usually in contact.

(d) A manuscript that is clearly acceptable on scientific grounds may nevertheless need certain changes in structure or improvements to the presentation. If the editor lacks either the time or the specialist knowledge to make these, a referee from the appropriate specialty can be asked for advice.

REFEREEING COMMISSIONED ARTICLES
OR CONFERENCE PAPERS

Everything that has been said here about refereeing unsolicited articles for journals applies in principle to other kinds of publication when referees are consulted, except that the editors must be much more forbearing with invited contributions than journal editors need to be with unsolicited manuscripts. For books, it is probably wisest to have only one, or at most two, advisers or consultants, to whom the editor can explain precisely what the book is aiming at: 'occasional' referees of odd chapters may produce a detailed but useless critique based on mistaken assumptions.

If journal articles, book chapters or conference papers which have been commissioned or accepted in principle seem on arrival to be unpublishable, editors certainly need advice, either to bolster their own opinions or to show them that their first impressions were mistaken. When a referee's guidance is requested in such a case, it should be made clear on which items the editor wants comments, but nothing should be said about the editor's particular misgivings if a truly independent opinion is wanted. If the referee confirms the editor's doubts, it is probably best if the contribution is rejected immediately; if the author is asked to revise the paper, a long and painful correspondence may be started which never leads to a satisfactory conclusion. Instead, the editor should write explaining that the contribution does not fit into the original conception of the book. If possible, some suggestions should be made about where else the paper might be published, so that the author does not feel that too much time has been wasted. Then, for journals or for books other than conference proceedings, another author can be invited to write an article or chapter on a similar but not identical subject, or the editor may write a chapter to fill the gap in a book—taking care not to plagiarize any of the rejected material! Tact, always an asset to an editor, as the next chapter implies, will have to be exercised if the author is not to feel wounded when the book is published.

REFERENCES

1. Ingelfiner, F.J. Peer review in biomedical publication. *American Journal of Medicine,* 56: 686-692, 1974.
2. Kochen, M. and Perkel, B. Improving Referee-selection and Manuscript Evaluation. In Balaban, M. (Ed.), *Scientific Information Transfer: The Editor's Role.* Boston, MA: D. Reidel Publ. Co., 1978, pp. 203-229.
3. Dyke, D.A. How I referee. *British Medical Journal,* 2:1117-1118, 1976.
4. Kochen, M. and Perkel, B., 1977, pp. 203-229.
5. Ingelfinger, F.J., 1974, 686-692.
6. DeBakey, L. *The Scientific Journal: Editorial Policies and Practices.* St. Louis: W.C. Mosby, Inc., 1976, pp. 12-13.
7. Neufeld, J. To amend refereeing (letter). *Physics Today,* 23:9-10, 1970.
8. DeBakey, L., 1976, pp. 18-19.
9. Pyke, D.A., 1976, pp. 1117-1118.
10. Prinz, G.A. More ideas on refereeing (letter). *Physics Today,* 23:11-12, 1970.
11. DeBakey, L., 1976, pp. 12-48.

"A Peerless Publication"

From E.P. Lewis, A peerless publication. *Nursing Outlook,* 28 (4): 225-226, May, 1980. Reprinted with permission.

Edith P. Lewis, R.N., recently retired from her position as editor of *Nursing Outlook*.

A Peerless Publication

by Edith P. Lewis

Today, from many corners of the academic nursing world, comes the call for the "refereed" or peer-reviewed journal. (While I have never seen the concept specifically spelled out, I assume it to mean a publication where the decisions about content are made by outside reviewers rather than by the editorial staff.) Hearing no similar call from other areas of nursing or from readers for such a system, I ask my friends in academia for their reasons. Their almost reflex response is, "more scholarly." When I press them to clarify what they mean by this, they then say; "Well, all the other disciplines in the university do it, and nursing has to be just as good as or the same as. . . ." While I do not personally subscribe to the refereeing concept save for certain selected journals, I believe it merits more than such a keeping-up-with-the-Joneses rationale.

First, one must ask, why do all the other disciplines "do it"? Probably because 1) it is the least expensive way to put out a journal which, in many cases, is subsidized by the professional organization and for which readers do not pay, usually receiving it as a membership benefit, and 2), more important, because there exists within the particular field a hard core of substantive knowledge against which the new submission can and should be judged.

The first reason would seem to have little relevance for nursing, but the second—the existence of a hard core of knowledge, methodology, or whatever—*is* valid for certain groups and journals within nursing, such as its research, scientific, or clinically specialized groups. Here I believe the refereed approach to be appropriate; it takes one expert to evaluate another's work. But to extend the concept to all of nursing's journals could, I believe, place a premature strait jacket on the exchange and expansion of nursing knowledge.

There is the risk, for instance, that a referee panel, once established, could turn into The Establishment—may, in fact, have been selected from its membership. I question neither the good intentions nor the expertise of the selected reviewers, but there *is* a human tendency to protect one's flanks against the upstart, the innovator, the challenger of givens. As Ingelfinger, writing about this in the May 1974 *American Journal of Medicine,* comments, it is possible that "the deviant approach, the maverick method or the totally new idea will not pass the censorship of the establishment." In a profession that has not yet agreed on even a definition of its nature, and in a publication like OUTLOOK that deals largely with trends, issues, and opinions, I believe the mavericks and the boat-rockers should have every opportunity to be heard.

In addition, how generally expert can the experts be? To the degree that they are selected because of their authoritative knowledge in the subject area represented by the magazine they serve, then one would expect a reasonable degree of inter-reviewer agreement. But, in the same article cited above, Ingelfinger reports that even for a specialized journal like the *New England Journal of Medicine,* the degree of reviewer concurrence proved to be only slightly better than might be expected by chance. There is no reason to think that the situation might be different in nursing, as attested to by those nurses who have received their papers back with totally different judgments from the individual reviewers. One might as well toss a coin—or leave it to the editors. This does not impugn the experts; it simply underlines the soft and fluid state of nursing knowledge.

It is interesting, I think, that the refereeing concept was initially characterized as peer review. But as one looks at the panel listings, it is evident that the "peer" has given way to the "authority" concept. Thus, the assistant professor, for instance, must write to please those above her in the educational hierarchy, although academic standards for a good paper are not necessarily the same as editorial ones for a publishable paper. Furthermore, she is likely to write not out of any motivation to share information with her colleagues, but because, if she wants to move up the academic ladder, she must publish. And, for the publication to count in some universities, it must be in a refereed journal. The noose tightens.

In fairness to my friends in academia (if I still have any), I should say that not all of them are pushing for the refereed idea; several, in fact, have encouraged me to open this discussion of it. And some others shrug their shoulders helplessly and say, "I know, I know— but that's the way it is in our university, and nursing has to go along." But the sheer number of nurses who are both writing and reading makes it difficult for nursing's publications to "go along" accordingly, for the logistics of the operation are formidable.

It boggles my mind, for instance, to think of, first, whiting out all identifying data, then making three photocopies of each of the approximately 500 manuscripts submitted to OUTLOOK each year, selecting the reviewers and sending the copies on to them, awaiting and collating the returns, and then doing whatever the reviewers advise doing! Moreover, the process would considerably delay both the decision about the paper and its publication; the innovative, fresh paper in 1980 may be old hat in 1982. Well, to hurry things along, it has been suggested, the editors could screen out the poor ones. But if they have the authority to screen out what they perceive as the poor ones, they may be tempted to screen in what they perceive as the good ones. After all, as someone once pointed out to me, the reviewers don't usually know who among them has evaluated which manuscript or what they have recommended. Any such fudging, it seems to me, diminishes the integrity of the editors, the presumably refereed journal, and the concept of refereeing itself.

What I find most disturbing is the uncritical acceptance of the "refereed is best" philosophy in a profession that places such a premium on validation of all its processes. Validation, within this context, would call for data proving that the refereed journal does indeed serve its readers better than the nonrefereed one. Is there objective evidence, for instance, that the content of the refereed journal is more informative, more useful, more responsive to readers' needs and interests (the ultimate test) than the nonrefereed one? To the best of my knowledge, there is no such evidence; more appalling, no one seems even to have looked for any. The refereed journal, for many, is taken as an article of faith, in the interests of academic respectability.

At this point, it is logical to ask: What makes judgments by an editorial staff any more valid than judgments by an outside review panel? With the proviso that these editors are well-qualified members of the profession served by their publication, then I would say that the answer is a combination of accumulated editorial wisdom, an open mind, and accountability to readers. Editors are exposed to a wide variety of current thinking, as represented by the many manuscripts that cross their desk and by the feedback, formal and informal, that they receive in great quantities; they develop a sensitivity to what is timely, important, authentic, and useful; they have no vested interests in any one school of thought, any one way of doing things; and I suspect that their scrutiny of papers is often more thorough than can be provided by the volunteer reviewer, trying to find time to read manuscripts in addition to her full-time job responsibilities. I would humbly suggest that just as there is research and clinical expertise in nursing, so, too, there is editorial expertise. And I'm not just talking about putting in the commas.

The smartest thing, though, about professional editors is that they know when they need help. OUTLOOK will soon be making formal its longtime informal practice of seeking outside consultation on manuscripts that we do not feel qualified to judge or when we feel the need for an outside opinion. But I, for one, see these external reviewers as consultants, not final authorities. I further believe the selection of content should be determined not by whether it meets the standards of a referee group, but whether it meets the informational needs of the readers—and I am convinced that editors know more about readers than anyone else does. It is my further contention that the referee concept, with its emphasis on "this is the way to earn brownie points for promotion and tenure," serves the interests of only one segment of nursing and not the interests of nursing and publishing as a whole.

It is possible, of course, that the refereed journal concept may render both me and my convictions obsolete.

FOR THE REFEREED JOURNAL

From H. K. Grace, For the refereed journal. *Nursing Outlook*, 28 (7): 423, July, 1980.
Helen K. Grace, R.N., Ph.D., is dean, College of Nursing, University of Illinois at the Medical Center, Chicago.

For the Refereed Journal...

by Helen K. Grace

OUTLOOK's April editorial ("A Peerless Publication") attributes the trend toward refereed journals to academia and a "keeping up with the Joneses" phenomenon. While the major push toward refereed journals is undoubtedly from academia, I hope that the concept is not discounted as having no applicability to nurses in other areas of practice. First, for those nurses employed in academic settings or those who wish to pursue academic careers, publications in refereed journals are an essential component of evidence necessary for gaining promotion and recognition in the academic world. While we may argue the pros and cons of this form of recognition, the reality remains that this is the way in which scholarly work is judged.

Nursing as a profession has fought a long and valiant battle to move nursing education out of the control of hospitals and into the academic mainstream. If we are to be a valid part of higher education, the standards by which we are to be judged are those inherent within this larger framework. Nurses developing careers in academic nursing are consistently penalized because there are so few nursing journals that have a well developed review process. Nurses, having invested a great deal of energy in preparing and submitting articles for publication, find that their efforts have been to little or no avail because the journals in which they have published are not refereed. Therefore their work is discounted. Were these journals refereed, it is most likely these very same articles would have been acceptable for publication. The nurse would then receive her rightful recognition.

While the above argument is based solely upon pragmatic considerations, the other issues raised in the editorial are of even greater concern. The argument that nursing lacks the "existence of a hard core of knowledge, methodology, or whatever" that other fields supposedly have is problematic and demeaning. It is through the very process of scholarly communication and exchange that this knowledge base is built. What is lacking in nursing publications is lively debate that serves to clarify issues and move the field forward.

In the editorial it is argued that a peer review mechanism would bring control over the field that would be undesirable. It is stated that a professional editor is better able to make judgments about what should be published than would a peer review group of nursing colleagues. In arguing these issues, there arises an area of some concern. Nursing is a marvelously diverse discipline. The practice domain of nursing must receive comparable attention to the research and theory domain, and hopefully there is congruence between the two. Nurses prepared at the doctoral level have come out of a variety of scientific disciplines and therefore they have competing points of view about the subject matter of nursing and how a knowledge base is to be built. It is extremely important in our review processes that this diversity be accentuated rather than repressed. It is essential that there be forums for expression of all points of view.

It is my personal belief that opportunities for publication of diverse points of view can be emphasized by a lively peer review process. A particular problem today is the stifling of the creative process in the way which most of our nursing journals "police" what is to be published.

I am not troubled by the number of new nursing journals that are being published. Given the size and diversity of the nursing profession and the multiple publics within this group, it is important that new avenues for points of view currently not expressed in the nursing literature be aired. It is through healthy competition that vigorous new ideas will be brought forth into the profession as a means of revitalization and growth.

"BOOK REVIEWING"

by L.E. Sissman

At some point in your career a journal editor may ask you to review a new book. Usually such a request concerns material in your area of expertise and the editor provides you with guidelines regarding the review's format. Thus the assignment may seem fairly straightforward and simple.

However, reviewing another person's book should be perceived as a weighty task; for the outcome of years of work as well as future career opportunities rest to a large extent on the reviewer's published opinion. Sissman's article, although focused for the literary reviewer of new fiction, contains solid advice that professionals reviewing other professionals' work should keep in mind. In specific terms he points out reviewers' obligations to themselves, to the authors they review, to their editors, and to their readers.

Book Reviewing
by L.E. Sissman

After years of stumping and (I hoped) dazzling other people with anything I cared to try in verse, at the hoary age of forty I became a book reviewer. Now it was my sworn and bounden duty to penetrate and unravel the obscurities of other writers' methods and messages, to dissipate the wet and inky smokescreen in which the wily squid conceals himself, and to set the delicate skeleton of the author's true design in so many words before my readers. Besides being hard, grueling detective work, this was both scary and risky; armed only with a shaky analytic gift and my spotty, idiosyncratic store of reading, I was laying my sacred honor on the line each time I tried to pick another literary lock in public.

For the first couple of years, I drove myself to write reviews like an aristocrat driving himself to the gallows, with superficial sangfroid as thin as onionskin and a real clutch of fear each time I sat down at the typewriter.

Then, mercifully, I began to learn the ropes and look a little more objectively around me. I discovered that reviewing was not simply something that a *soi-disant* literary man did to fill time, amplify his tiny reputation, and (of course) earn a little money. *Au contraire.* Reviewing, it was slowly and astoundingly revealed to me, was a vocation, a craft, a difficult discipline, with its own rules and customs, with a set of commandments and a rigid protocol. Mostly by making painful mistakes and leaping brashly into pitfalls, I began to amass some notion of the shape of a reviewer's obligations to himself, to the author he reviews, to his editor, to his readers.

In short, I became aware of the moral imperatives of book reviewing. Funny as that may sound in a literary world raddled by cliques and claques and politics, by back-scratching and back-stabbing, by overpraise and undernotice, I now believe that the would-be conscientious reviewer must be guided by a long list of stern prohibitions if he is to keep faith with himself and his various consumers. In the interests of controversy (and, I hope, of air-clearing), I set these down herewith.

1. Never review the work of a friend. All sorts of disasters are implicit here; a man and his work should be separate in the reviewer's mind, and the work should be his only subject. If you know the man at all well, you become confused and diffident; your praise becomes fulsome, and you fail to convey the real merits and demerits of the book to the poor reader. The hardest review I ever wrote was of the (quite good) novel of a friend four years ago. Never again.

2. Never review the work of an enemy. Unless you fancy yourself as a public assassin, a sort of licensed literary hit man, you will instinctively avoid this poisonous practice like the plague it is. Corollary: never consent to be a hatchet man. If Editor X knows you are an old enemy of Novelist Y, he may (and shame on him, but it happens all the time) call on you to review Y's latest book. Beware, on pain of losing your credibility.

3. Never review a book in a field you don't know or care about. Once or twice I've been touted onto titles far from my beaten track. The resulting reviews were teeth-grindingly difficult to write and rotten in the bargain. Unless you're a regular polymath, stick to your own last.

4. Never climb on bandwagons. You are not being paid to subscribe to a consensus, nor will your reader thank you for it. If a book

has been generally praised (or damned), you add nothing to any-body's understanding by praising (or damning) it in the same terms. Only if you have read the book with care and found something fresh to comment on should you attempt a review. Otherwise, find some-thing else (how about the work of an unknown?) to write about. Or skip it; you'll earn that money you need for a new 500mm mirror lens somewhere else.

5. Never read other reviews before you write your own. This is a tough rule to follow, because all reviewers are naturally curious about the reception of Z's latest book. Nonetheless, you can't help being subtly influenced by what *The New York Times* reviewer (or whoever) has to say. Eschew!

6. Never read the jacket copy or the publisher's handout before reading and reviewing a book. Jacket copy (I know, I used to write it) is almost invariably misleading and inaccurate. The poor (literally: these downtrodden souls are, along with retail copywriters, the most underpaid people in advertising) writer is probably working from a summary compiled by the sales department, not from a first-hand reading of the book. The handouts are more of the same, only flackier.

7. Never review a book you haven't read at least once. Believe it or not, some reviewers merely skim a book (or even depend on, horrors, the jacket copy) before reviewing it. Not only is this a flagrant abdi-cation of responsibility; there is always the lurking danger of missing a vital clue in the text and making a public spectacle of yourself. It should happen frequently to all such lazy reviewers.

8. Never review a book you haven't understood. If *you* haven't figured out what the author is up to, there's simply no way you can convey it to your reader. Reread the book; if necessary, read some of the author's other books; if you still don't know, forget it. The cardi-nal sin here is to go right ahead and condemn a half-understood book on the covert grounds that you haven't found its combination.

9. Never review your own ideas instead of the author's. Unless you're the ranking pundit in the field and you have a scholarly bone to pick with the author, you have no right to use the book under inspection as a springboard for a trumpet voluntary of your own.

10. Never fail to give the reader a judgment and a recommenda-tion on the book. And tell why. A reviewer is really a humble con-sumer adviser; his main job is to tell the public what to read and what

to skip. It's an important job because nobody can possibly keep up with all the books being published today.

11. Never neglect new writers. First novelists, in particular, get passed over too frequently for several reasons. The obvious reason is that Norman Mailer's new novel is better copy than Hannah Furlong's maiden effort. The less obvious reason is that it's much harder for a reviewer to get an intelligent fix on an unknown. In short, it's harder work to review a debutant.

12. Never assume that a writer is predictable. This is, in a way, the converse of the previous proposition. Part of the pleasure of picking up a new book by a writer you've read before is *knowing* what you're about to read—the themes, the style, the old, familiar tricks. But what if the novelist has *grown;* what if he does something daring and unexpected? That's when a lot of reviewers, myself included, are tempted to put him down for not rewriting himself. The only answer is to approach the book with great caution and read it on its own merits, forgetting what has gone before.

13. Never forget to summarize the story or the argument. What's more maddening than a review that rhapsodizes (or bitches) for two thousand words about the author's style, his technique, his place in letters without ever giving us a clue to the nature of the story, beyond the mention of an incident or two?

14. Never, on the other hand, write a review that is merely a plot summary and nothing more. This happens surprisingly often, especially in newspaper reviews. The reader of the review deserves a judgment, a rating, not simply a recapitulation.

15. Never impale a serious writer on his minor errors. Nobody's perfect, as the old gag line says, and, given the susceptibility of even the most powerful piece of work to ridicule, it is frighteningly easy for the reviewer to have his fun at the author's expense and end up distorting the value and import of the book. (Example: I recently read a good novel in which the author consistently misused the word "fulsome" and mixed up "she" and "her." It would have been an act of willful irresponsibility to take the author to task for these small miscues, which were also his editor's fault.)

16. Never write critical jargon. The day of the New Criticism, for all its good, is mercifully past, and so, I'd hope, is the compulsion of some reviewers to pose and posture as anointed gospelers of the true and beautiful. The reviewer who writes for a general-circulation

newspaper or magazine should have his typewriter unplugged if he persists in pedagogeries.

17. Never fail to take chances in judgment. Because it forces you to enter the mind of another on his own terms, reviewing is literally mind-expanding. Often the reviewer is astonished at his new conclusions and afraid to put them down on paper. This is a mistake; one of the highest critical acts is to arrive at a new understanding and communicate it to the reader.

18. Never pick a barn-door target to jeer at. Not long ago, one of the daily reviewers in *The New York Times* wasted an entire column on the new novel by one of the Irving Wallaces. Irving Stone? Jacqueline Susann? Or whoever. Anyway, it was painfully easy— shooting fish in a barrel—and painfully unworthy of the reviewer's taste and talent. He might far better have reviewed a good first novel.

19. Never play the shark among little fishes. Being a reviewer does not entitle you to savage the beginner, the fumbler, the less-than-accomplished writer. A sincere and decent effort demands a sincere and decent response. If you've ever struggled to write a book yourself, you know the vast amounts of pain and love it takes. To put down an honest attempt in gloating arrogance is to deal a crippling blow to a nascent career of possible promise.

20. Never compete with your subject. A reviewer is not, at least during his hours as a reviewer, a rival of the person he's reviewing. If he sees flaws in the work under inspection, he should report them, but he should not give vent to a long harangue on how *he* would have written the book. (If his hubris is that keen, perhaps he should take time off and write a book himself.)

In a word, then, the sins and temptations of reviewers are legion. As an incumbent sinner, I have more often than I like to think about been brought up short by the realization of my own weaknesses. Thus the list above. While I know I don't have the constancy and fortitude to follow it to the letter, I try to bear it in mind, like a catechism, when I sit down to write about another person's work. It is the least I can do for another poor sufferer who has taken the supreme risk of letting his dreams and talents go forth between covers, and for all those poor sufferers who simply like to read, and who rely, for better or worse, on the dim and uncertain skills of reviewers for a guide through the maze of new titles in their bright, unrevealing jackets on the shelves.